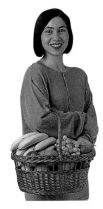

HEALTH AND HEALING
THE NATURAL WAY

THE HEALING
POWER OF FOOD

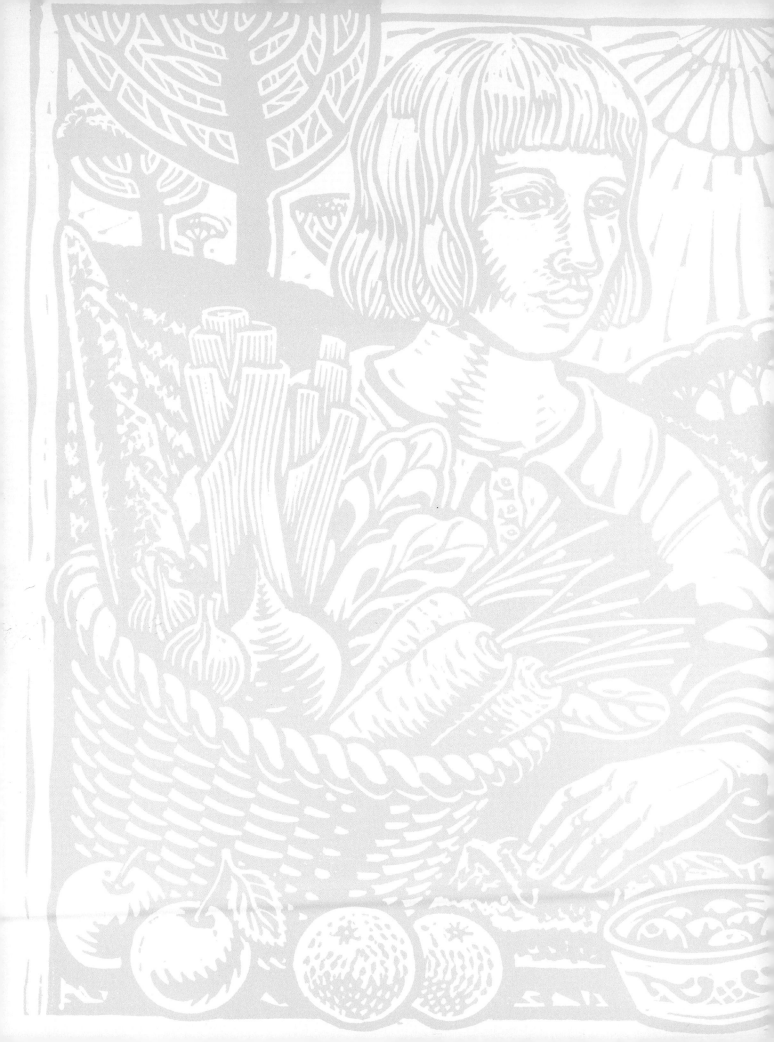

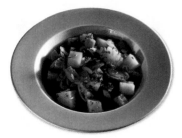

HEALTH AND HEALING
THE NATURAL WAY

THE HEALING POWER OF FOOD

Reader's Digest

PUBLISHED BY

THE READER'S DIGEST ASSOCIATION, INC.

PLEASANTVILLE, NEW YORK / MONTREAL

A READER'S DIGEST BOOK
Produced by
Carroll & Brown Limited, London

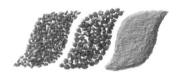

CARROLL & BROWN

Publishing Director Denis Kennedy
Art Director Chrissie Lloyd

Managing Editor Sandra Rigby

Editor Laura Price
Assistant Editor Joel Levy

Art Editor Adelle Morris
Designer Simon Daley

Photographers Jules Selmes, David Murray

Production Christine Corton, Wendy Rogers

Computer Management John Clifford

First English Edition Copyright © 1997
The Reader's Digest Association Limited,
11 Westferry Circus, Canary Wharf,
London E14 4HE

Reprinted with amendments 1998

ISBN 0-7621-0260-8

Printed in the United States of America
Second Printing, August 2000

SENIOR CONSULTANT

Dr. Alan Stewart MBBS, MRCP

NATUROPATHY CONSULTANT

Roger Newman-Turner
BAc, ND, DO, MRO, MRN

RECIPE CONSULTANT

Jane Griffin BSc (Nutrition), SRD

CONTRIBUTORS

Sian C. Porter BSc (Hons), SRD
Nicola Seabrook BSc, SRD
Anita Bean BSc
Linda Lazarides BA (Hons)
Maria Pufulete
Jill Scott
Natalie Field BSc, SRD

READER'S DIGEST PROJECT STAFF

Project Editor Gayla Visalli
Editorial Director, health & medicine Wayne Kalyn
Design Director Barbara Rietschel

READER'S DIGEST ILLUSTRATED REFERENCE BOOKS, U.S.

Editor-in-Chief Christopher Cavanaugh
Art Director Joan Mazzeo
Operations Manager William J. Cassidy

The information in this book is for reference only;
it is not intended as a substitute for a doctor's diagnosis and care.
The editors urge anyone with continuing medical problems
or symptoms to consult a doctor.

Address any comments about *The Healing Power of Food* to Editor
in Chief, U.S. Illustrated Reference Books, Pleasantville, NY 10570

THE HEALING POWER OF FOOD

More and more people today are choosing to take greater responsibility for their own health rather than relying on their doctor to step in with a cure when something goes wrong. We now recognize that we can influence our health by making certain improvements in lifestyle—eating better, doing more exercise, and taking measures to reduce stress. People are also becoming increasingly aware that there are other healing methods—some new, others ancient—that can help to prevent illness or be used as a complement to orthodox medicine.

The series *Health and Healing the Natural Way* can help you make your own health choices by giving you clear, comprehensive, straightforward and encouraging information and advice about methods of improving your health. The series explains the many different natural therapies now available, including aromatherapy, herbalism, acupressure, and a number of others, as well as the circumstances in which they may be of benefit when used in conjunction with conventional medicine.

The approach of THE HEALING POWER OF FOOD is to emphasize the direct medicinal effects that can be achieved with food. It explains the general principles of healthy eating, how diet relates to disease, and exactly how the active components of food work. The main thrust of the book is, however, to provide clear, practical guidelines on what to eat to relieve a wide variety of health problems.

THE HEALING POWER OF FOOD reflects the growing trend to bring alternative therapies and mainstream medicine together. The book does not seek to challenge orthodox medical practice but rather to complement it with healthful eating practices. To this end the benefits of foods are presented within the context of a well-balanced diet that can help you achieve optimum health.

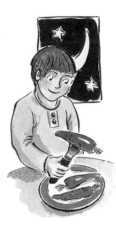

CONTENTS

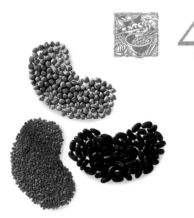

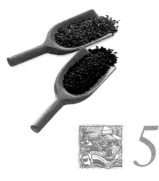

5 Managing illness with food

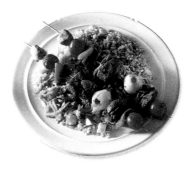

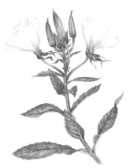

6 Plans for Health

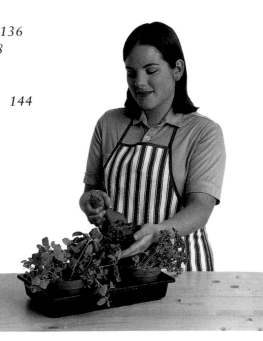

A HEALTHY DIET

With an understanding of the vital role food plays in health, longevity, and fighting disease, you may regard your daily meals in a completely new light.

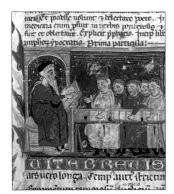

HIPPOCRATES
(c.460–370 B.C.)
Generally regarded as the father of Western medicine, Hippocrates included much dietary advice in his writings. The medieval illustration above shows Hippocrates.

MEDITERRANEAN FOODS
The Mediterranean tradition of cooking and eating has descended from the ancient Greeks and Romans, with a few later additions, such as the eggplant.

Until recently, the role of a balanced diet has been greatly misunderstood and misapplied. With infectious disease largely conquered by modern medicine, degenerative disease has become the Western world's primary killer, and an inexorable tide of research and statistics shows that poor diet is among the biggest contributors to these disorders. This is not the poor diet of failed crops or drought. Instead, inadequate diets in the West are brought about by ignorance, the time pressures of hectic lifestyles, and the growing dependence on fast foods and prepackaged meals. Many people do not seem interested in the benefits of fresh foods and a well-balanced diet, and general health is failing as a result.

Mainstream medicine, which for many years denied or overlooked the role of diet in good health, is at last coming round to much older ways of thinking about balanced diets and, more specifically, to recognition of the direct medicinal powers of some foods. Nutritional cures that have come down to us through history are now being combined with a modern understanding of their effects and are finding new acceptance.

5,000 YEARS OF EATING FOR HEALTH

Some of the earliest written records demonstrate cultural beliefs in the healing properties of foods and practice of herbal and nutritional remedies. Both the ancient Egyptians and the Sumerians advocated the benefits of a variety of medicinal plants that we still use today. The Egyptians used honey for treating wounds and skin problems and aloe vera as a sun block. The ancient Greeks were renowned for dispensing medical and dietary advice. Pythagoras, the Greek scientist and philosopher, was an evangelical vegetarian, while Hippocrates, the father of Western medicine, recommended wheat and barley brans for their laxative effects.

The Romans further dispersed this store of knowledge; various encyclopedias written between the 1st century and 4th century A.D. were enormously influential on European dietary practice for the next 13 centuries. Their advice was sometimes wrong—Galen, for instance, warned against eating fresh fruit—but the Roman Empire did pass on a fondness for salads, which lasted through the Middle Ages and up to the Enlightenment. In 1699 John Evelyn, a charter member of the Royal Society, wrote a whole book on the marvelous properties of salads, particularly the "soporifous [sleep-inducing] qualities" of lettuce.

SCIENCE OVER NATURE

Beginning in the early 18th century, medicine began to turn its back on herbal cures and to elevate science over nature. Exceptions like James Lind's discovery of the link between citrus fruit and scurvy were rare, and herbal and dietary cures were left to the quacks and faddists. This didn't make them any less popular. Zeal for the dietary route to good health peaked in the 19th century when the American Sylvester Graham first made popular the belief that diet was the determining factor in health and claimed that whole-grain bread was the panacea for all modern ills. He was followed by the cult figures of James H. Salisbury and John Harvey Kellogg, whose followers were told that indigestion caused every disease, from typhoid to mental derangement.

Meanwhile, scientists were hard at work uncovering the biology of nutrition. As early as 1825, William Prout had identified proteins, carbohydrates, and fats as the major components of food, and almost 90 years later the first vitamin, naturally named A, was discovered. Despite such advances, mainstream medicine showed little interest in using these discoveries or investigating the health-giving properties of food until the counter-culture movement of the 1960s, with its emphasis on back-to-nature principles and concern for the environment, awoke a new curiosity about natural cures. Since then the slow buildup of interest in alternative therapies and holistic approaches to medicine has encouraged a willingness to put nutritional medicine to the test. Gradually many of the old traditions have proved to be grounded in scientific fact and have been percolating back into the mainstream.

NEW WORLD VEGETABLES
European colonization of the New World introduced new vegetables—including potatoes, tomatoes, and peppers—to Europe, adding to the many native varieties and those brought from Asia in ancient times. Until the 18th century most vegetables were grown only in private gardens for personal consumption.

JOHN EVELYN (1620–1706)
Known mainly for his Diary, *Evelyn was also an ardent admirer of salads. In 1699 he wrote* Acetaria: A Discourse of Sallets.

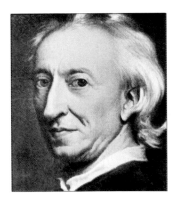

OLD TRADITIONS LIVE ON

In much of the world, however, the old traditions never lost their followers. Chinese and Indian Ayurvedic medicine, for example, are based primarily on herbal lore and treatments, many of which have been or are under investigation in the West. Ephedrine, used to treat asthma, derives from the ancient Chinese remedy ma huang (ephedra), while artemisia, used to treat fevers in China for 2,000 years, is being hailed as a new weapon in the fight against malaria. Ginger for nausea and honey for its laxative effect are also important food curatives in oriental medicine.

Honey is popular around the world, recommended for everything from minor skin wounds to sore throats to insomnia. Aloe vera is still used in Africa today as a salve for wounds and burns. Yogurt is a favorite remedy in Mediterranean countries for many types of infections and digestive problems, and garlic is considered a cure-all almost everywhere it is found. In fact, folk medicine here and abroad has a use for almost all the herbs, vegetables, and fruits that we use today, and more has been forgotten than herbalists will ever know.

UNDER THE MICROSCOPE

There is a steadily lengthening list of drugs used in mainstream medicine that have been developed from herbal or folk remedies. Quinine, from the South American cinchona plant, is a well-known example, while serious scientific studies have backed up several therapeutic claims made for ginger, garlic, onions, fish oils, and a host of other food products.

General practitioners in some European countries now routinely prescribe food-based treatments for common disorders. German doctors advise garlic capsules for hypertension and high levels of blood cholesterol; the antiemetic properties of ginger are being harnessed to combat chemotherapy-induced nausea; and fatty acids from fish oils and soy protein are components of a new HIV drug.

THE ENEMY WITHIN

Our understanding of how food helps the body overcome adverse conditions has been radically altered by new insights into molecular biology. A picture of the day-to-day workings of our cells has emerged, and it shows that the single greatest threat to our health may actually be the natural waste products of ordinary metabolism.

FISH OIL, GINGER, AND GARLIC
These commonplace food-stuffs have joined the front line in the fight against disease. The therapeutic value of fish oil is a relatively recent discovery. Ginger and garlic, on the other hand, have been used as curatives since ancient times, but are only now coming into their own as proven health aids.

When the microscopic machinery of the cell uses oxygen to break down food molecules like complex carbohydrates, fat, or protein and thus release energy, highly reactive molecules are created as by-products. These molecules, called free radicals, are also created by a variety of other agents, such as cigarette smoke, pollution, sunlight, and viruses. Once loose in the body, they can damage cell membranes, proteins, and particularly DNA—the molecule that carries all the genetic information about a living organism. Damaged DNA can give rise to faulty cell function, so when the cell reproduces, it may be incorrectly copied or even divide erratically, thus leading to cancer. Free radicals have also been implicated in atherosclerosis, the clogging of arteries with cholesterol.

Normally, free radicals are mopped up by antioxidants, and any DNA damage is quickly repaired. But under conditions of stress, exposure to damaging substances like cigarette smoke or pollution, illness, or dietary deficiencies, the ability of the body to cope with free radicals is compromised. Over time, damage builds up, leading eventually to degenerative disease or cancer.

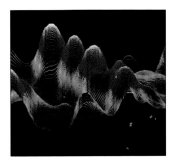

DNA UNDER FIRE
DNA, shown here as a color-enhanced electron micrograph with the coils of its double helix visible in the center of the image, carries the blueprint for all our bodily processes and structures. Any of them can suffer when free radicals cause damage to DNA.

THE SECRET INGREDIENTS OF FOOD

Scientists are discovering that fruits, vegetables, grains, and legumes are a treasure trove of antioxidants and substances with antioxidant-enhancing properties. These plant chemicals have been collectively termed phytochemicals, and more than a dozen different classes have been discovered. How they work is often unclear, but they seem to be most effective in their natural form, that is, as part of a whole food rather than an artificial supplement.

Many animal products also contain health-promoting antioxidants. Their vitamins and minerals, especially zinc, selenium, and manganese, are all effective against free radicals and in boosting the body's immune system and self-repair mechanisms.

The burgeoning science of nutrition has uncovered many substances in addition to antioxidants that promote well-being. The omega-3 fatty acids found in fish oils help protect against heart disease by lowering cholesterol levels in the blood and also thinning it, thus preventing dangerous clots from forming. There is growing evidence also that they can soothe the painful effects of arthritis and psoriasis. Allicin, the substance that gives garlic its characteristic odor, has the same effect. Garlic also contains antibacterial and antiviral substances. The role of dietary fiber has

WHEN TO BEGIN
Healthy eating should not be something you turn to when you leave school, start a family, or retire, but should be with you all your life. It's never too late, however, to benefit from a healthy diet.

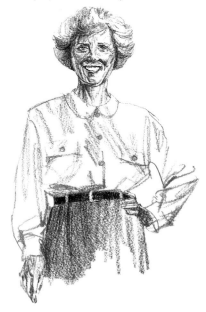

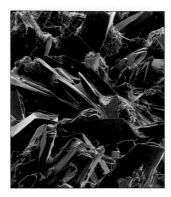

GLUCOSE CRYSTALS
The basic product in the breakdown of carbo-hydrates—glucose—shown in the micrograph above, is the energy that drives our bodies. Low levels of glucose, indicated by lethargy and tiredness, may be caused by metabolic disorders. (See chapter 5.)

SHOPPING FOR HEALTH
Healthful food is not necessarily expensive, especially when you shop for fresh foods in season.

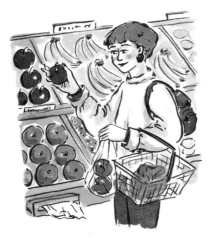

been found to be an important one in both protection against and relief from many digestive disorders. Fiber, provided by many plant foods, promotes digestion and bowel movements. It also helps protect the body from several types of cancer, particularly cancer of the colon, while the form known as soluble fiber, plentiful in apples, beans, and the bran of certain grains such as rice and oats, helps reduce cholesterol.

ARMING YOURSELF FOR THE FIGHT AGAINST ILL HEALTH

In order to take advantage of nature's wealth of healing chemicals, you need to understand the components of a healthy diet and be able to identify the areas where your own food intake might be lacking. Armed with this knowledge and the guidelines set out in this book, you can start to target specific maladies or disorders and actually treat them with your diet.

The Healing Power of Food takes you through the basics of nutrition, starting with the general principles, next focusing on individual foods and conditions, and finally presenting integrated dietary programs for common conditions. Chapter 1 presents an overview of food and its relation to overall health and reviews advancements in nutritional science. Chapter 2 looks at disease and food in general, while chapter 3 details the healing components of many specific and diverse types of food.

Once the essentials of nutrition and its relation both to health and disease have been set out, chapters 4, 5, and 6 move on to more specific concerns. Chapter 4 describes a comprehensive range of healing foods, detailing how they work, what they prevent or treat, and how to choose, store, prepare, and serve them. Chapter 5 systematically examines major illnesses, diseases, and disorders and explains general and practical aspects of dietary therapy for each. Finally, chapter 6 presents a range of fully integrated dietary and lifestyle programs to help you deal with some of the most important health issues of today, from quitting smoking to treating irritable bowel syndrome.

Throughout the book special features describe some of the major therapeutic approaches in the field, and case studies illustrate practical issues about the treatment of disorders related to diet. A comprehensive glossary completes the picture, providing a valuable and clear reference to help you become and stay healthy with foods.

DO YOU NEED HEALING FOODS?

Perhaps you already treat a bout of the flu with a bowl of chicken soup, and you may believe that boosting vitamin C intake can help with a cold. But few people are aware of the incredible range of health benefits that good food can bring or the impact that the wrong diet can have on physical and mental well-being.

Q **IS YOUR DIET BALANCED?**
Perhaps the central tenet of all dietary advice should be that balance is essential. Using food as medicine is not about sudden bingeing on a particular vegetable or fruit or drinking tomato juice with every meal. Apart from becoming bored, you could miss out on a variety of substances, from essential fatty acids and vital vitamins to complete proteins and trace minerals; you could even end up with a severe deficiency. In order to target a specific disorder, you need to eat a fully integrated and balanced diet that meets all your needs. To find out what an imbalanced diet could be doing to your body, see chapter 1 and learn how to eat for good health.

Q **DO YOU KNOW WHAT SUPERFOODS ARE?**
If your knowledge of nutrients extends only as far as the back of your breakfast-cereal box, you might be amazed to find out just how much natural power to prevent or cure disease is contained in the simplest of foods. Did you know that whole-grain bread contains not only complex carbohydrates but also fiber, protein, vitamin B_1, iron, and niacin? Or that salmon provides iodine, fluoride, selenium, zinc, iron, and omega-3 fatty acids? Chapter 4 details the natural pharmacy contained within hundreds of different foods.

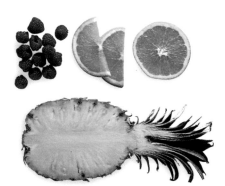

Q **DOES YOUR FAMILY HAVE A HISTORY OF ILLNESS?**
Disorders like osteoporosis, diabetes, and high cholesterol levels, even the risk for some forms of cancer, can be hereditary. You may be resigned to suffering from similar problems, but careful control of your diet, along with proper medical care, may produce startling results in the prevention, management, and cure of many such conditions. See chapters 2, 5, and 6 for specific dietary advice on individual disorders.

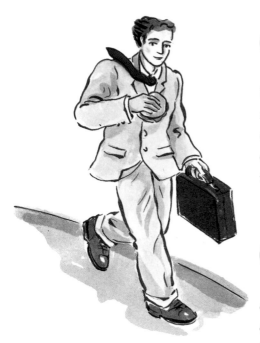

Q DO YOU SKIP MEALS OR EAT ON THE RUN?

People very often skip breakfast or lunch, perhaps as part of a deliberate attempt to keep their weight down or possibly because a busy lifestyle allows no time to eat. But the damage done by missing regular meals can far outweigh any reduction in calories. Losing out on essential nutrients can weaken your immune system, and if your energy supply is irregular and fitful, you could end up tired for most of the day. Chapter 1 explains just what you miss when you skip a meal.

DO YOU OFTEN FEEL TIRED OR LACKING IN ENERGY?

Q If you find that you are often tired and lethargic, it could be your diet that's to blame. To maintain your metabolism at its proper levels, you need to supply the cell machinery with a balance of essential nutrients. For example, the efficiency of your blood as an oxygen carrier may be compromised if you are not eating enough iron-rich foods such as meat, fish, poultry, beans, and dried fruit. Lack of the B vitamin folate also contributes to anemia; whole grains and fortified cereals are good sources of this important nutrient. See chapter 6 for an energy-restoring plan to help you make dietary and lifestyle changes that will boost your energy levels.

Q DID YOU KNOW THAT BRAN CAN BE BAD FOR YOU?

The benefits of bran—the coating of cereal grains often removed in the milling process—are numerous. It helps prevent constipation, promotes a feeling of fullness (an aid to weight loss), may reduce the risk of some kinds of cancer, and in the case of oat and rice brans, helps lower blood cholesterol levels. However, too much bran can aggravate inflammatory bowel disease or cause diarrhea, and the phytic acid in raw bran prevents absorption of such vital minerals as calcium, iron, zinc, and magnesium. Chapter 4 has more information about cereals.

Q DID YOU KNOW THAT ALCOHOL CAN BE GOOD FOR YOU?

The negative aspects of alcohol, which include its toxic effects and the fact that it is high in calories—empty ones, at that—are well documented. However, numerous studies have shown that in moderation, alcohol can be beneficial. In fact, wine, especially red wine, is believed to be one of the components of the Mediterranean diet that protects against heart disease. See chapter 4 for additional details.

CHAPTER 1

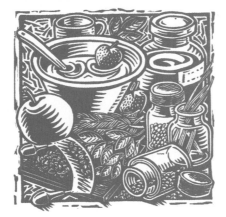

FOOD AND YOUR HEALTH

Let food be your medicine and medicine be your food. *—Hippocrates (c.460–370 B.C.)*

Many familiar foods have roles as preventative or healing agents. In past times and other cultures, this idea was commonly accepted, but then the growth of technological medicine pushed the healing role of food into the background in developed countries. Now it is enjoying a renaissance.

FOOD AS MEDICINE

A number of medicines used for preventing or treating common conditions are derived from sources more usually accepted as foods.

WELL-KNOWN REMEDIES

Some of the folk remedies handed down from generation to generation involve food.

▶ *Ginger for nausea*

▶ *Cloves for toothache*

▶ *Peppermint for indigestion*

▶ *Honey for a sore throat*

▶ *Prunes for constipation*

▶ *Carrots for night vision*

▶ *Citrus fruit and garlic for a cold*

▶ *Parsley for bad breath*

CARROT VISION
Carrots are an excellent source of vitamin A, a deficiency of which has long been linked with eye problems, particularly night blindness.

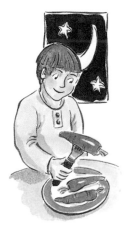

The medicinal properties of plants have been recognized and put to use since the beginning of civilization. Even today herbal remedies are thought to make up as much as three-quarters of all medicines taken around the world. In Western countries many traditional plant remedies are being investigated by scientists to determine if they have beneficial effects and, if they do, to identify the active ingredients that produce these results.

One example of a food used as medicine is rhubarb, the stalks of which are best known as an ingredient in puddings and pies. Its roots and rhizome have been used around the world in the treatment of both constipation and diarrhea.

Furthermore, many drugs have been derived from molds that grow on foods. The antibiotic penicillin was originally made from bread mold, and ergot, a mold that grows on rye, is used in the treatment of postchildbirth hemorrhage and migraine. Other food molds are being used to treat fungal infections.

SCIENTIFIC RESEARCH

Derivatives of plants have saved thousands of lives. Rosy periwinkle, for example, was traditionally used in Madagascar for the treatment of diabetes. Trials by the drug company Eli Lilly in the 1960s found no evidence that it worked for this purpose, but when the pure extract was administered to laboratory rats with tumors, scientists noticed that it had an anticancer effect.

Research into a means of controlling or curing HIV and AIDS has included a close look at food-based derivatives. A special food, Advera, has been developed for use by patients with HIV and AIDS. It is high in omega-3 fatty acids and contains a unique soy protein, fiber, beta carotene, and other vitamins and minerals.

REMEDIES AROUND THE WORLD

Cultural differences in diet and medicinal uses of food are now being investigated by modern researchers because epidemiological studies (research into the causes and distribution of diseases affecting a population) show that certain populations have a greatly reduced or increased risk of developing particular diseases. Studies by the World Health Organization, for example, have revealed a clear connection between diet and heart disease in a number of countries (see chapter 2).

Regional remedies

Climate and geography play a large part in determining the diet and food remedies of a region and its culture. For example, people who live along the Rhine River in Germany are at higher risk for rheumatic disorders because of their damp environment, but they also have a plentiful supply of willow trees, which grow by water. The bark and leaves of willows were traditionally used to treat rheumatic pains. Extraction of salicin, the active pain-relieving ingredient in the willow, led to the development of a synthetic version, acetylsalicylic acid, which is better known as aspirin,

Practitioners of folk medicine in India use plants of the genus *Coleus* to treat various ailments, from indigestion to fever. Tubers of these plants are also used for adding spicy flavors to food. One variety, which contains forskolin, reduces intraocular pressure and is prescribed in the United States to treat glaucoma. More research is underway to find additional commercial uses for these plants.

Ephedra, known as ma huang in China and squaw tea in North America, has been traditionally used to treat asthma, allergies, and colds. Its active ingredient, ephedrine, is a nasal decongestant. The herb is also a potent nervous system stimulant that in excessive doses can cause nervousness, headache, palpitations, and other effects. When it was discovered in the early 1990s that ephedra increases the rate of metabolism, thus helping people on weight-loss diets to burn more calories, many abuses occurred and some people even died from overdoses. Since then, warnings have been issued about the dangers of ephedra, and in Canada only government approved ephedrine products are considered safe for use.

The juice of aloe vera was employed in ancient Greece as a cure-all. Cleopatra applied it as a sunscreen. Africans use it for burns and wound healing; the Chinese use it as a laxative. In Europe it is now commonly incorporated in various skin products.

Honey, another favorite remedy of ancient Egyptians, was used for treating wounds and skin problems. Around the world honey has been recommended for diarrhea, coughs, sore throats, and insomnia. South African tests have shown promising results using honey for bacterial infections in the gut.

Chinese healers have used ginger for motion sickness for centuries. Today ginger is being tried out for use in treating pre- and post-operative nausea, as well as nausea caused by chemotherapy.

Other traditional remedies under scientific inspection include an infusion, or tea, made of 10 plant materials that are commonly used in Chinese medicine for the treatment of skin problems. Controlled clinical trials have shown that this brew produces a short-term beneficial response in people who are suffering from atopic eczema.

The garlic remedy

Garlic, considered to be a cure-all in many different cultures, has been under extensive scrutiny by today's medical researchers, with impressive results. The active ingredient of garlic, allicin, which is responsible also for its characteristic odor, has been found to reduce blood cholesterol, lower blood pressure, and inhibit clot formation in the blood. Work continues to determine if garlic actually reduces the frequency of and mortality from heart disease.

DISEASE PREVENTION AND FOOD

Many people are aware of the work carried out by James Lind in the 18th century that led to the identification of scurvy, caused by vitamin C deficiency, and its cure with citrus fruit—two oranges and a lemon daily.

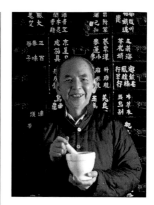

OLD AND NEW
Practitioners of Chinese medicine have long understood the powers of plants and herbs in healing. They use the majority of such plants in their natural state, either the dried leaves and flowers or the root, and advocate making them into teas or chopping and adding them to foods.

HEALING APPLICATIONS

Although interest in the medicinal use of food is growing all the time and many applications may appear to be innovative and new, most cultures have long histories of food-based remedies. Some of these remedies have never dropped out of use, and many have now been scientifically proven to have beneficial health effects. The foods below are used either in their natural state or in recognizable man-made concentrations of their active compounds, which are available as tablets, powders, or creams.

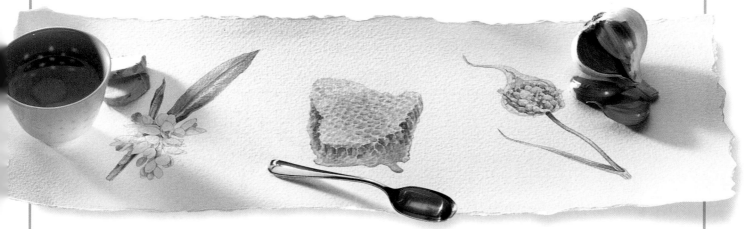

Ginger Linked today with reducing the inflammation of arthritis, ginger also relieves nausea and is recommended to alleviate the symptoms of colds and influenza.

Honey In the West we know honey best as a soothing treatment for sore throat and cough, but it has also been used to treat minor skin wounds and inflammations.

Garlic The antifungal and antibacterial properties of garlic are well known, but it also reduces high blood pressure, high cholesterol levels, and relileves gastrointestinal ailments.

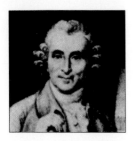

JAMES LIND
British physician Lind became a major figure in naval health reform, instigating delousing procedures and the use of hospital ships.

FOOD AND DRUG INTERACTION

Invariably, the label on a prescription or over-the-counter medicine will give instructions relating to the timing or the dose relative to eating: "Take half an hour before food;" "Do not take with milk." This is because foods can affect the absorption or action of a drug. In turn, drugs can affect certain nutrients in foods. Oral contraceptives, aspirin, and some antibiotics lower blood levels of vitamin C, for example.

The growing interest in the medicinal properties of foods is increasing people's awareness of the connection between food and health. It's best to consult your doctor, however, before treating yourself or seeking food remedies from alternative therapists for serious or persistent problems.

Origins

In the early 18th century, many sailors suffered from scurvy—painful sores and bleeding gums and mucous membranes—during long voyages. Dr. James Lind observed that there was a link between the incidence of scurvy and the lack of fresh fruits and vegetables in the sailors' diets. We now know that they were suffering from severe vitamin C deficiency.

Although Lind recommended that citrus fruit be issued to sailors, it was years before the British Navy ordered them to take one lime a day; hence their nickname "limeys."

More recently a longer life expectancy has been linked to a diet rich in all fruits and vegetables (see pages 58–64).

Numerous trials are currently being done to determine the role of certain nutrients, and the foods rich in these nutrients, in protecting against and preventing disease. For example, lycopene, a carotenoid found in tomatoes, is being studied for its antioxidant properties. Other products being examined for antioxidant effects include onions, tea, and red wine.

FOOD AS MEDICINE TODAY
In North America the role of food as medicine has been a neglected area in the medical profession. Doctors have primarily prescribed drugs or suggested surgical procedures and have often been unaware of the possible health benefits of certain foods. This attitude is now changing, but there is still some way to go.

In many European countries the idea of food as medicine is already more widely accepted. In Germany, for example, garlic capsules are prescribed by medical practitioners for hypertension (high blood pressure) and to help reduce cholesterol, yet in this country they are available only in health food stores for self medication.

In recent years, however, many people have become skeptical about pharmaceuticals and there is growing support, backed by research, for managing some illnesses with natural remedies. The alternative, or complementary, medicine of food is slowly gaining mainstream acceptance. Some health practitioners now recommend using

fish oils to relieve rheumatoid arthritis and eczema and to prevent heart disease. A study from the *Lancet* in 1985 showed a reduction in joint tenderness and morning stiffness in patients with rheumatoid arthritis after taking fish oil supplements for 12 weeks. Other studies have shown that a regular diet of oily fish significantly improves the cardiovascular health of heart attack survivors, protecting them against further attacks.

Some areas of medicine have been using diet in disease management and treatment for some time. For example, non-insulin dependent diabetes is treated in many cases with diet alone; adhering to a diet high in fiber, low in fat, free from refined sugar, and with a moderate alcohol intake keeps blood sugars at normal levels. The diet of patients with kidney disease is essential to their treatment, so much so that eating too much of the wrong foods—those high in protein, salt, and phosphorus, for example—could be fatal. Consequently, all renal patients regularly see a dietitian for monitoring. General practitioners also refer patients to dietitians for a wide variety of chronic problems, such as skin disorders and allergies.

THE ANTIOXIDANT PROTECTOR

Foods high in antioxidants, which protect the body against the damaging effects of free radicals, can easily form part of a balanced diet.

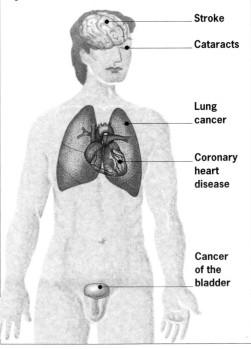

Stroke

Cataracts

Lung cancer

Coronary heart disease

Cancer of the bladder

FOOD AND HEALTH

A balanced lifestyle and diet are necessary to achieve and maintain good health and prevent disease. Deficiencies or overconsumption can put you at risk.

A healthful diet is one that contains nothing harmful and supplies adequate but not excessive amounts of required nutrients and calories. In theory, this should be relatively simple to achieve, given the wide choice of foods available, but with choice comes the problem of eating more than you should of a particular food because you like it or it is convenient rather than because you need it.

AN UNHEALTHY DIET
Although most people associate deficiency diseases with famine-stricken populations, they also occur in conditions of plenty. Many busy people find it easier to blame their tiredness or inability to concentrate on too much work, the weather, or the time of year than a possible lack of iron. Because deficiencies are not always obvious, often they are not detected until they are relatively advanced. Other problems result from eating more than the body needs.

Eating disorders
Two of the most severe eating disorders in the West are anorexia nervosa and bulimia, psychological conditions based on a distorted body image and fear of being fat. Sufferers of anorexia starve themselves, while those with bulimia habitually binge and follow their binges with vomiting or purging. Both conditions may result in severe nutritional deficiencies.

Iron deficiency
Maintenance of iron levels in the body depends not just on how much iron is present in the diet but also on how well it is absorbed by the body. Absorption of iron in the digestive system,

especially iron from plant foods, is improved by the presence of vitamin C and reduced by other substances, such as the tannin in tea and the caffeine in coffee. If you are trying to increase your iron level, it is recommended that you drink orange juice with an iron-rich meal and avoid drinking tea or coffee for at least two hours afterward to maximize absorption. A combination of poor dietary intake of iron and increased need, during pregnancy, for example, or during growth spurts, can lead to iron-deficiency anemia. Symptoms include physical and mental fatigue and an increased incidence of illnesses such as colds and flu.

Protein-energy malnutrition
A deficiency of protein and lack of energy are closely linked. Protein-energy malnutrition, in which insufficient protein leads to low

ABSORBING IRON
To achieve optimum absorption of iron, combine foods that contain this valuable mineral (those on the left, below) with foods high in vitamin C (those on the right). The richest suppliers of iron are meat, shellfish, whole-grain breads and cereals, and dried legumes. Modest sources include eggs, dried fruits, peas, and parsley.

Who needs supplements?

Most people do not need or benefit from supplements. There are some exceptions, however.

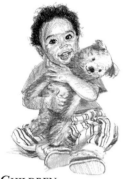

CHILDREN
Picky eaters may need vitamin and mineral supplements.

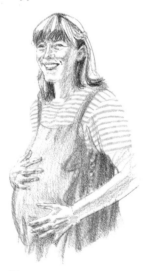

PREGNANT WOMEN
Mothers-to-be may be advised to take extra folate, iron, and calcium.

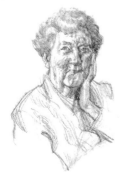

THE ELDERLY
Elderly people who are infirm have special needs for supplements.

energy, is currently the most widespread form of malnutrition, affecting more than 500 million children and adults worldwide, mostly but not exclusively in poorer areas. The effects of inadequate food intake are poor growth in children and weight loss and wasting in adults.

In the affluent West, protein deficiency is usually found only in conjunction with some underlying problem such as cancer, inflammatory bowel disease, alcoholism, or an eating disorder such as anorexia nervosa. It may also be a side effect of chemotherapy or radiation therapy, which are used to treat cancer. Extreme poverty, lack of education, and social isolation can also contribute to protein deficiency.

IS FOOD ENOUGH FOR HEALTH?

There has been a lot of debate as to whether vitamin or mineral supplements are necessary or if food alone can supply all the nutrients a healthy person needs. Overwhelming evidence points to the fact that a balanced diet is the best way of obtaining all the recommended nutrients for optimum health.

The liver, which stores vitamins and minerals, makes up for occasional dietary lapses by releasing them. And when the body is given more vitamins and minerals than it needs through supplementation, it generally excretes them in the urine. However, several vitamins and minerals are hazardous in high doses. For example, doses of vitamin C above 1,000 mg a day can increase the risk of kidney stones and cause bladder irritation. In high doses vitamin A can cause liver damage, skin problems, and fatigue. Excessive amounts of vitamin D can lead to calcium deposits in the heart and blood vessels and upset calcium metabolism, eventually leading to bone loss.

The role of supplements

Some people *are* more at risk of developing nutritional deficiencies than others. Supplements can help people with specific needs maintain necessary nutrient levels when it is difficult to achieve these levels through diet.

Your diet is probably adequate if you are not in any of the at-risk groups described below and regularly meet the healthy eating guidelines given on page 24. If you are concerned about the possible health risks of your diet, ask your doctor to refer you to a dietician or nutritionist.

WARNING

Some supplements greatly exceed the recommended levels, and certain vitamins and minerals taken in megadoses can cause nutritional imbalances, even become toxic. For example, excessive amounts of zinc can cause nausea, diarrhea, even death if taken in doses that build up in body tissues.

The institutionalized

Anyone who depends on a residential institution for nutritional needs can be at risk of deficiencies. The often strict budgets of hospitals, homes for the elderly, prisons, and schools can lead to limited food choices and meals that are overcooked, unattractively presented, and not well balanced.

A prime example of deficiency risk would be poor vitamin C intake because of a low consumption of fresh vegetables and fruits, or lack of vitamin D because of being housebound through illness.

Young children

A pediatrician may recommend vitamin and mineral supplements for children who are very poor eaters or chronically ill. It is important that these be geared to the child's age and weight to avoid overdosing.

Pregnant women

For women who are pregnant or planning pregnancy, experts recommend a daily intake of 4 mg of folic acid (see page 28)—the amount in seven servings of broccoli. Supplements may be helpful in meeting this requirement. This group may also need more of other nutrients, including vitamin D, calcium, and iron. But caution is advised because excessive amounts, particularly of vitamins A and D, can harm the fetus.

Acutely and chronically sick

People with severe or chronic illnesses are at increased risk of deficiencies because of such factors as poor appetite, drug-nutrient interaction, and malabsorption. They may therefore need to take supplements.

Voluntarily restricted diets

Groups in this category include vegetarians, particularly vegans, and those on strict weight-reduction or elimination diets. They

Using a Food Diary to

Watch Your Health

If you have a health problem, it could be food related. Taking note of how you feel after eating can highlight elements of your diet that might be causing ill health and suggest changes that might benefit both your short- and long-term well-being.

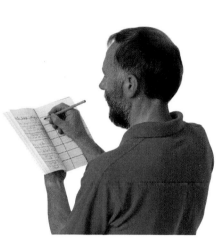

The first step in making a connection between your diet and health is to keep a food diary. Write down everything that you eat or drink, including quantities and cooking methods. Don't forget sugar in hot drinks or oil used for cooking. Each day, note where, when, and why you ate the food and how you felt before and after. Also record any ill feelings you had, when they occurred, and how long they lasted.

After two weeks, look back over your diary and see if you can identify any connections. Did a headache come on after drinking coffee, for example, or a rash break out after you consumed certain dairy products?

If you identify a problem food, eliminate it from your diet for a week or two and monitor the effects. Then gradually reintroduce it and note any changes in health. Check the labels of foods you eat: hidden ingredients or their by-products can sneak into your diet and upset your experiment.

If problems persist, see your doctor or a qualified nutritionist and help this person to assist you by relating the details of your food diary.

KEEPING A FOOD DIARY
Any health problems related to the foods you eat can be sorted out rapidly once you have identified the problem foods. Noting the foods you consume over a two-week period will help. Be sure to include drinks and garnishes; it might be the raw onions on your salad that are giving you indigestion.

POINTS TO CONSIDER

It may help to expand your food diary into a diary of general health. You can note other aspects of your life that may affect your health and try to see if they are related to or worsened by your diet.

▶ *Are you taking any medication? It could contribute to symptoms.*
▶ *Have you been sleeping properly? Could this be related to your diet?*
▶ *Are your hair and skin in good condition? A well-balanced diet is crucial for healthy hair and skin.*

▶ *Are you having any emotional problems? These could affect your eating habits.*
▶ *If you are a woman, do you have problems with premenstrual syndrome? Some symptoms of PMS can be relieved with dietary changes (see page 112).*

INTOLERANCE TO DAIRY PRODUCTS

This is one of the most common of food intolerances. Dairy foods come in many forms, so be sure to eliminate them all if you want to test whether they are the cause of your problems. Remember to check food labels because dairy products can turn up in unexpected places.

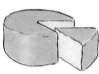

MILK
Look for milk in breads and other baked goods, also in packaged mixes.

CHEESE
You can find cheese and its by-product whey in dips, sauces, crackers, and icings.

YOGURT
Yogurt is often an ingredient in prepared dips, sauces, and cake mixes.

BUTTER
Check for butter and buttermilk in baked goods and creamy sauces.

CREAM
Keep an eye out for cream in pasta dishes and pastries.

CHANGING TIMES

One result of modern progress is that lifestyle and food are now risk factors in many disorders, such as cancer and heart disease. People select their food from supermarket shelves instead of hunting and gathering it. The result is a less healthy lifestyle for some, but a vastly improved one for others because of the varied selection of foods available all year long.

HUNTER-GATHERER
A physically active life produced strong muscles and cardiovascular fitness.

No pollutants or pesticides meant no allergic reactions to them and also life with fewer man-made carcinogens.

Natural, untainted foods meant no added sugar or salt in the diet, hence less obesity and fewer salt-related circulatory problems and strokes.

Sometimes poor, monotonous diet led to deficiencies, tooth and gum disorders, and bone problems.

Dependence on natural resources may have led to seasonal deficiencies, malnutrition, and starvation.

20TH-CENTURY MAN
Modern methods of food preservation and storage mean few, if any, dietary deficiencies.

A highly stressful lifestyle, coupled with insufficient periods of relaxation, may contribute to many illnesses and diseases.

A more sedentary lifestyle can lead to such problems as obesity and heart disease.

Dependence on high-fat, high-sodium foods can lead to many disorders, from skin complaints to heart disease.

Smoking tobacco and drinking alcohol can lead to cancer, liver problems, and heart and lung disorders.

risk missing out on certain nutrients that need to be replaced by taking supplements.

Others at risk

Women who suffer heavy blood loss during menstruation are at risk for iron deficiency. People who emigrate from African and Asian countries to the West often suffer dietary problems because of sudden and often dramatic changes in their diets. Also, anyone who smokes or drinks heavily is greatly at risk for deficiencies. Smokers, in particular, have reduced levels of vitamins A and C and calcium in their blood than nonsmokers.

CHANGING NUTRITIONAL NEEDS

Humans started out as hunter-gatherers and ate whatever they killed or picked in the wild. Stone Age humans probably consumed no alcohol and little added salt, and their only concentrated source of sugar was honey. Their diet was high in fiber and predominantly based on plants rather than animals.

Over time, humans have developed other methods of supplying their food needs, for example, by farming, by canning, freezing, and other processing methods, and by importing foods not grown or available locally. The result is a very wide dietary choice and availability.

Modern affluence means that people eat not only for nutritional purposes but also for pleasure, for social and business reasons, and out of boredom. These changes have not been balanced by a biological adaptation. Humans are still physiologically hunter-gatherers but now gather food in supermarkets and expend little energy in the process.

When people radically alter their diet, their body behaves somewhat like a car that has been designed to run on unleaded gasoline but is filled with leaded. It gives poor performance, becomes prone to problems, and may eventually break down altogether. Examples of this can be seen among southern Asians living in Western countries who have adopted a Western diet and have a much higher incidence of diabetes and heart disease than similar groups living in Asia. Similarly, liver disease and diabetes have risen dramatically in the oil-rich Arab countries over the last 50 years as increased wealth has changed people's lifestyle.

FOOD SENSITIVITY

Food sensitivity is a broad term used to describe allergies and food intolerances. As Lucretius (96–55 B.C.) elegantly summarized, "One man's meat is another man's poison." Although food sensitivity has been recognized for centuries, it is still a relatively new field in medicine and one that is full of confusion. This is partly because there is no simple diagnostic test for an allergy that compares with other diagnostic tools, such as measuring blood sugar levels for diabetes.

Allergies

Allergic reactions are caused by certain foods stimulating the body's immune system to produce antibodies, which in turn trigger production of histamine and other irritants and destructive substances that are released into the bloodstream. A specific allergy to food can be confirmed by tests. Symptoms may include vomiting, rash, and diarrhea.

A severe reaction can cause anaphylactic shock, which is characterized by difficulty in breathing, rapid pulse, profuse sweating, and collapse; in rare cases it can be fatal. If an allergy test is negative for a food that produces an adverse reaction, the problem is usually a food intolerance (see page 142).

Keeping a food diary

Keeping a diary of food intake and symptoms (see page 21) can help you identify a food intolerance or allergy. Sometimes an exclusion or elimination diet may be needed to confirm your suspicions. This approach involves removing suspect foods from the diet for a week or two, then reintroducing them while keeping a record of symptoms. Such a diet carries the risk of deficiencies. It is inadvisable to follow an elimination diet for a long period of time and without qualified supervision from a registered dietitian or your doctor.

Changes with age

Tolerance to foods can increase with age; for example, children who are unable to drink cow's milk may be able to tolerate it later in life. Conversely, you can develop sensitivity to a food that you have eaten all your life. For instance, some older people lose the ability to produce lactase, the enzyme needed for digesting cow's milk, and so can no longer tolerate dairy products.

Aversion to food

Food aversion is a psychological intolerance for certain foods. Sometimes people avoid a particular food because they think they cannot eat it or because it has unpleasant associations; for example, someone given ice cream during a hospital stay may always connect it with feeling unwell.

HIDDEN INGREDIENTS

It is essential to check ingredients lists very carefully if you are avoiding a particular food because it may be present under an unfamiliar name. Casein and whey, for example, are milk proteins. Dairy and corn products and eggs all appear under many different names.

▶ *Dairy products: casein and caseinate, whey, whey syrup sweetener, milk solids, butter, yogurt, cheeses*

▶ *Corn: cornstarch, corn oil, corn syrup, corn flour, cornmeal, corn-oil margarine*

▶ *Eggs: Dried eggs, egg albumin, egg lecithin, egg yolk*

ALLERGIES

An allergic reaction is an extreme or unusually severe response of the immune system to a substance that is usually harmless. When the body comes into contact with such a substance, or antigen, the immune system misidentifies the antigen and attempts to destroy it by producing antibodies and releasing chemicals that detect and attack the harmless element. One of these chemicals, histamine, can cause the sneezing (in hayfever), wheezing (in asthma), and hives (in food and drug allergies) that are typical allergic responses.

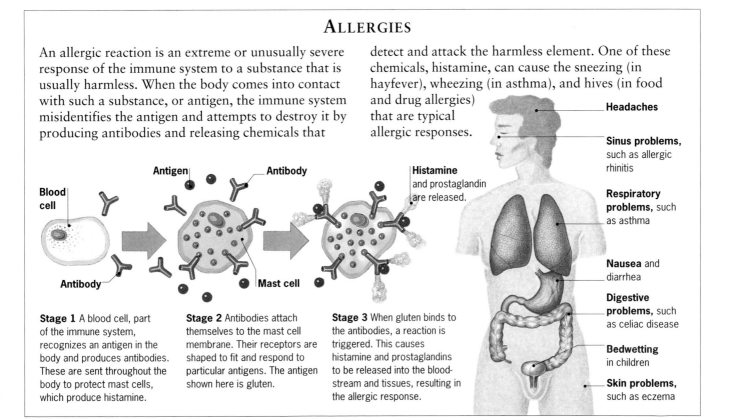

Stage 1 A blood cell, part of the immune system, recognizes an antigen in the body and produces antibodies. These are sent throughout the body to protect mast cells, which produce histamine.

Stage 2 Antibodies attach themselves to the mast cell membrane. Their receptors are shaped to fit and respond to particular antigens. The antigen shown here is gluten.

Stage 3 When gluten binds to the antibodies, a reaction is triggered. This causes histamine and prostaglandins to be released into the bloodstream and tissues, resulting in the allergic response.

Blood cell · Antigen · Antibody · Antibody · Mast cell · Histamine and prostaglandin are released.

Headaches

Sinus problems, such as allergic rhinitis

Respiratory problems, such as asthma

Nausea and diarrhea

Digestive problems, such as celiac disease

Bedwetting in children

Skin problems, such as eczema

BASIC HEALTHY EATING

The first step in using food to promote health and prevent disease is to establish a balanced eating plan that consistently includes all the nutrients your body needs.

BALANCING ACT
An easy-to-remember approach to a diet that contains the right balance of foods is the 1-2-3-4-5 plan. Each day you eat one serving of meat, fish, poultry, eggs, or a combination of legumes or nuts and grains, two of milk or milk products, three of fruits, four of vegetables, and five of bread and other starchy foods. Eat fats and sugars sparingly.

The secret to maintaining a healthy diet, one that contains all the essential nutrients you need, is to eat a variety of foods in the right proportions. One simple way of doing this is to follow the plan described at the left.

HEALTHY EATING GUIDELINES

The general guidelines below apply to most people, but age, activity levels, illness, or pregnancy can create different needs. If you have any questions or concerns about the effects that your diet may be having on your health, speak to a doctor or a registered dietitian or nutritionist, who can give you advice on how to make adjustments.

Fruits and vegetables

If you follow the 1-2-3-4-5 plan, you will be eating seven servings of fruits and vegetables every day. This may seem like a lot (most people meet about half this quota), but it is fairly easy to double portions of each food you select to fulfill the requirements. Examples of servings are ½ cup of cooked vegetables, 1 cup of raw leafy greens, 1 medium-size apple, ¾ cup (6 ounces) of fruit juice, and ½ cup of diced fruit.

Whenever possible, do not remove edible skins because these are high in nutrients and dietary fiber. Take advantage of seasonal specials to obtain the freshest and most flavorful produce, and vary your choices and methods of preparation to experience different textures and flavors.

Raw fruits and vegetables make ideal snacks because they are low in fat and calories (with the exception of avocados). Most are also high in fiber, which makes them filling and therefore satisfying.

Fruits and vegetables have the added health benefit of being high in antioxidants, which help protect against many diseases by preventing damage from the free radicals that are formed in the metabolic process.

Starchy foods

Complex carbohydrate, or starchy, foods include bread, rice, pasta, cereals, and other grain products. Some nutritionists include the potato in this group because of its high starch content, although it is technically a vegetable with a good vitamin C content not found in grains. Ideally, you should eat at least one portion of a starchy food with every meal, and altogether complex carbohydrates should form the bulk of your overall eating plan. Examples of servings are 1 slice of bread, ½ cup of cooked pasta or rice, and 1 ounce of dry cereal.

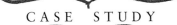
A Vegan

A vegan diet, which does not contain any animal products at all, can be very healthful. Vegans have to be more careful than the average person, however, to balance plant foods in such a way that they provide sufficient amounts of the protein, vitamins, and minerals that most people obtain from meat, fish, poultry, and dairy products.

Jill is a 21-year-old management trainee for a large pharmaceutical company. She lives alone and has been a vegan since the age of 12. Having been on a strict vegetarian diet for so long, Jill is confident that she knows how to balance her meals to obtain all necessary nutrients, and she often buys take-out vegetarian dishes at a local eatery. Still, Jill has been constantly tired lately, has been having repeated bouts of colds and flu, and is prone to acne. Her doctor has sent her for various tests, but these have not revealed any problems except borderline anemia, for which he has prescribed iron supplements. Thinking that she may have some deficiencies in addition to iron, Jill has decided to consult a nutritionist.

WHAT SHOULD JILL DO?

For at least two weeks before visiting the nutritionist, Jill should keep a food diary, noting everything she eats and when. On her own, she could start to evaluate her diet by comparing the vitamins and minerals she receives through her diet with the recommended dietary allowances. By not doing much of her own cooking, she may be losing the opportunity for a better balance of nutrients. Her fatigue and repeated illnesses may be symptoms of deficiencies in zinc and/or vitamin B_{12}, as well as iron. The nutritionist is also concerned that Jill may not be getting enough calcium. Stress on the job could be causing Jill's acne and be a factor in her lowered immunity; she should find ways to relax.

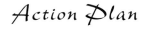

Action Plan

DIET
Eat more citrus fruits to aid the absorption of iron from vegetables and beans. Include more zinc-rich foods, such as legumes, nuts, and whole-grain breads. Add more dark leafy greens for calcium.

STRESS
Reduce stress levels by making time each day for yoga exercises or meditation.

EATING HABITS
Set aside time each week for planning menus and make sure that the kitchen is stocked with necessary supplies.

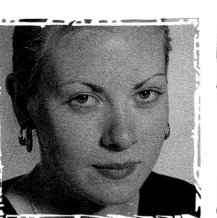

DIET
The secret of a healthy vegan diet lies in balancing a variety of different foods.

EATING HABITS
Depending too much on take-out foods can lead to deficiencies of some nutrients.

STRESS
A very stressful lifestyle can lower immunity and cause unpleasant physical symptoms.

HOW THINGS TURNED OUT FOR JILL

Once Jill understood that her health problems were partly related to her diet, she started making weekly menu plans and doing more of her own cooking instead of relying on take-out dishes. She also signed up for yoga classes to help her control the stress produced by her job. On the advice of the nutritionist, Jill began taking supplements of vitamin B_{12}, zinc, and calcium, as well as iron. Her skin is now clear of blemishes and she has energy to burn.

Like fruits and vegetables, small amounts of starchy foods make good snacks. These help keep up energy levels without the often negative side effects encountered with sugary or caffeinated foods.

To make the most of starches, choose whole-grain varieties and prepare or serve them with as little fat as possible. You can use vegetable-based rather than meat- or cream-based sauces for pastas. Also, spread margarine or butter sparingly on bread to keep your fat intake to the recommended limit of 30 percent of daily calories or less.

Protein foods

This food group includes meat, shellfish, fish, poultry, and eggs, all of which provide complete proteins, that is, all the essential amino acids that the body needs but cannot manufacture itself. The recommended total intake of such high-protein foods is about 6 ounces per day. As a percentage of daily calories, protein should comprise 10 to 15 percent.

Legumes, nuts, and seeds are also high-protein foods, but they are not complete unless combined with grains. Typical combinations include lentils and rice, baked beans and corn bread, pita bread with hummus (chickpea–sesame seed spread), pasta with fava beans, and peanut butter on toast. Combinations can be eaten at the same meal or at different meals on the same day.

While nuts are a good source of protein, they are also high in fat. Fortunately, most of their fat is in monounsaturated or polyunsaturated, and does not clog arteries the way saturated fats in animal foods do.

Milk and dairy foods

Dairy products are an important source of protein, B vitamins, and calcium. Low-fat and nonfat varieties have just as many nutrients as whole-milk products and are the best choices for adults who want to limit their intake of fat. They are not suitable for children younger than five, however; youngsters

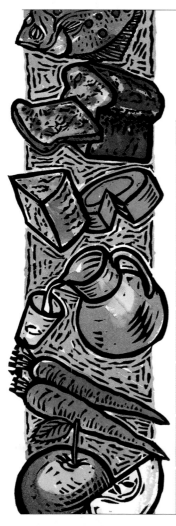

COMPONENTS OF A HEALTHY DIET

The various elements in foods that make up a healthy diet are listed below. All are essential for normal bodily function, and deficiencies in any can cause illness.

It is important to maintain a balance, incorporating the best amounts of each group to achieve and maintain the healthiest diet possible.

NUTRIENT	FUNCTION	GOOD SOURCES
Protein (amino acids)	Is essential to growth and repair of tissues; helps regulate many chemical processes in the body.	Meat, seafood, eggs, milk and cheese, soy products, legumes, nuts, grains
Fat	Provides energy (calories); supports hormone production; aids absorption of fat-soluble vitamins—A, D, E, and K.	Butter, margarine, vegetable oils, meat, fish, whole-milk dairy products
Carbohydrate	Converts readily to glucose, the body's main source of energy.	Bread, pasta, rice, cereals, legumes
Dietary Fiber (a nonstarch polysaccharide)	Promotes elimination; soluble type may lower cholesterol levels.	Whole-grain bread, pasta, and cereals; brown rice; potato skins; fruits and vegetables
Vitamins	Varies according to specific type; in general, essential to all vital processes in the body.	Fruits, vegetables, animal foods, starchy foods
Minerals	Varies according to specific type; in general, vital for keeping body cells energized, bones and teeth strong.	Vegetables, fruits, animal foods, starchy foods, milk products; some water
Water	Is important for all bodily functions.	All foods and beverages

VITAMINS AND MINERALS

Most foods contain vitamins and minerals to a greater or a lesser degree. The aim is to achieve the ideal intake of those nutrients that you most need for optimal health. A balanced diet will usually provide them without the need for supplements.

NUTRIENT	ESSENTIAL FOR	SIGNS OF DEFICIENCY	GOOD DIETARY SOURCES
Vitamin A	Growth; reproduction; healthy skin; good vision	Night blindness; dry skin; stunted growth in children	Liver, oily fish, orange and yellow fruits and vegetables
Vitamin D	Healthy bones	Rickets; tetany; osteomalacia	Fortified margarine, milk, and butter; egg yolks; oily fish
Vitamin C	Wound healing; healthy connective tissue, teeth, and gums	Scurvy; sore gums; poor wound healing; easy bruising	Citrus fruits and juices, berries, peppers, broccoli, tomatoes, potatoes
B_1 (Thiamin)	Normal digestion, appetite, and nerve function	Muscle weakness; brain and nervous system dysfunction	Milk, meat, poultry, yeast, whole-grain cereals, beans
B_2 (Riboflavin)	Healthy skin	Fatigue; sore mouth; vision problems	Milk, green vegetables, meat, fortified cereals
B_3 (Niacin)	Normal metabolism and growth; large amounts can lower cholesterol.	Diarrhea; dermatitis; digestive problems; mental disturbance	Eggs, meat, seafood, poultry, fortified cereals, brown rice, yeast, legumes
B_6 (Pyridoxine)	Protein metabolism	Dermatitis; depression; anemia; painful nerve endings	Fish, meat, poultry, green vegetables, fortified cereals
Folic acid	Healthy red blood cells; protein formation; DNA synthesis	Anemia; neural tube defects, such as spina bifida	Green leafy vegetables, dairy products, fortified cereals
B_{12}	Healthy red blood cells; protein and fatty-acid metabolism	Anemia; painful nerve endings	Meat, poultry, shellfish, fish, eggs
Vitamin E	Antioxidant	Unknown in humans	Vegetable oils, margarine, green vegetables, nuts, cereals, eggs, seeds
Vitamin K	Normal blood clotting	Poor blood clotting	Leafy green vegetables, liver, pork
Calcium	Healthy bones and teeth; cell-to-cell communication	Bone diseases such as rickets, osteomalacia, osteoporosis	Dairy products, green leafy vegetables, fish with bones
Phosphorus	Healthy bones and muscles; cellular energy metabolism	Muscle wasting; respiratory failure; nerve degeneration	Cereals, meat, poultry, fish, eggs, dairy products, nuts
Magnesium	Protein synthesis; bone, nerve, and muscle development	Muscle weakness; rapid heart rate; loss of appetite; cessation of menstruation	Meat, nuts, cereals, beans, green vegetables
Iron	Hemoglobin production; immune function	Anemia	Liver, meat, fish, poultry, fortified cereals, legumes
Zinc	Wound healing; normal growth; sexual development	Growth retardation; impaired healing; immune dysfunction	Meat, fish, shellfish, whole-grain cereals, eggs
Copper	Body processes; absorption of iron	Low white blood cell count; increased risk of infections	Liver, fish, shellfish, fruit, green vegetables
Iodine	Thyroid hormones, which regulate metabolic rate	Goiter	Seafood, milk, some cheeses, eggs, iodized salt

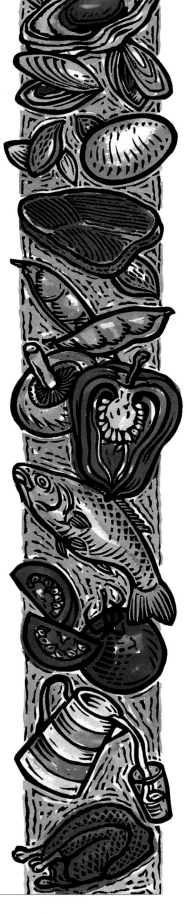

need the fat from whole milk for growth. One serving equals an 8-ounce cup of milk or yogurt or 1½ ounces of cheese. Women and children, in particular, need to make sure they are getting enough calcium.

Vegans can use soy milk enriched with calcium and vitamin B$_{12}$, as well as tofu and other soy products, to meet their dairy needs. People who are lactose sensitive (allergic or intolerant to milk and milk products) can also use enriched soy milk, or they can try goat's milk, lactose-reduced cow's milk, or yogurt, which has only one-third to two-thirds of the lactose usually found in milk.

Fatty foods

Fats are necessary to health. They contribute to growth, production of sex hormones, and maintenance of cell membranes; provide energy; and aid in absorbing the fat-soluble vitamins—A, D, E, and K. Fats also stimulate the intestines to release a hormone that suppresses the appetite and thus signals us to stop eating. Surprisingly, the fat needed in our diet is minuscule, about one tablespoon per day of polyunsaturated fats containing the essential fatty acids linoleic acid and linolenic acid, neither of which can be manufactured by the body. If we limited ourselves to such a small amount, however, our meals would be much less satisfying. On the other hand, many people obtain up to 40 percent of daily calories from fat, which is far too much. About 30 percent is the recommended maximum, with no more than 10 percent of daily intake from saturated fats.

Sugary foods

Foods made with a high percentage of refined sugar are not needed in a healthful diet; their calories are largely empty ones, and they are a major cause of tooth decay. When eaten as snacks, sugary foods provide an immediate rush of energy that burns off just as quickly as it came. Despite such drawbacks, sugar unquestionably brings pleasure, satisfies an inborn taste for sweets, and in small amounts is harmless in an otherwise well-balanced diet.

Recommended dietary allowances

In the United States the Food and Nutrition Board of the National Research Council, a branch of the National Academy of Sciences, proposes Recommended Dietary Allowances, or RDAs, for 11 vitamins, 7 minerals, and protein, and lists the estimated safe and adequate intakes of two other vitamins and five minerals. These allowances, considered adequate to meet the nutritional needs of healthy people, are reassessed and updated every 5 to 10 years.

To determine a specific RDA, nutrition scientists establish a minimum amount, below which deficiency develops, and a maximum, above which toxicity or other damage might occur. The RDA falls between these two values, thus creating a margin of safety for periods when there may be insufficient intake and allowing for individual differences in absorption of nutrients. In general, it is not necessary to fulfill RDAs on a daily basis. They are meant as guidelines by which you can assess whether your diet comes up to healthful standards.

Because foods vary in the types and amounts of nutrients they contain, a widely varied diet based largely on grains, fruits, and vegetables and small amounts of high-protein animal foods, plus a limited intake of fats and sugar, is the best way to achieve and maintain good health.

FOLIC ACID

Folic acid, also known as folate or folacin, is a B vitamin essential to making DNA, RNA, and red blood cells. During pregnancy it helps prevent certain neurological defects.

From 1983 to 1991 the Medical Research Council in the United Kingdom conducted a trial involving 1,195 women who had previously had a baby born with spina bifida or other neural tube defect. The trial showed that a folate supplement of 4 mg per day for three months prior to conception and for the first three months of pregnancy reduced the risk of having another baby with a neural tube defect by 75 percent. Subsequently a much smaller dose was shown to be effective.

In the United States the daily recommended dietary allowance of folate for pregnant women is 400 mcg daily; 180 mcg is the RDA for all other women and girls. Because the most critical period for folate consumption is during the first 4 to 6 weeks of pregnancy, some physicians believe that all females of childbearing age should routinely take a folic acid supplement.

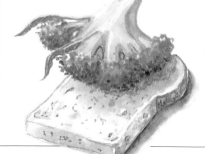

DIETARY SOURCES OF FOLATE
Good natural sources of folic acid include broccoli, dark green leafy vegetables, lentils and other dried legumes, citrus fruits, and fortified breads and breakfast cereals.

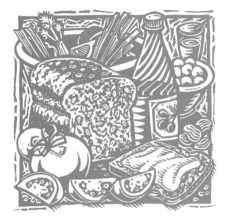

CHAPTER 2

PREVENTING DISEASE WITH FOOD

It is becoming increasingly clear that there is a strong relationship between diet and the incidence of many diseases that plague our society, such as cancer, heart disease, and stroke. Some diseases can be prevented entirely by nutritional measures, while the chance of developing others can be greatly reduced by eating the right foods, even if other factors are present.

NUTRITION-RESPONSIVE DISEASES

In the Western world some of the most widespread disorders are directly related to nutrition and can be partially or completely prevented or treated by dietary measures.

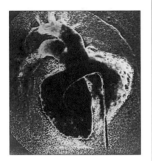

DIET VERSUS GENES
Many disorders, such as high blood cholesterol, heart disease, and high blood pressure, have a strong genetic component. But a genetic tendency does not make these problems inevitable. With good eating habits and regular exercise, it is possible to maintain a healthy body and beat your genes.

Admittedly, some inherited diseases, like sickle cell anemia, and many congenital disorders, such as the hole in the heart shown above, cannot be influenced by diet. But other problems, including low birth weight and spina bifida, are directly related to the diet of the mother.

Heart disease and some forms of cancer are just two examples of diseases for which diet is known to play a central role. And many other conditions, from celiac disease and migraine headaches to constipation and obesity, respond well to changes in diet. Sensitivity to certain foods can also result in illnesses of varying seriousness. These can be treated by dietary changes that involve replacing the problem foods with different ones.

DIGESTIVE PROBLEMS
Constipation is a common problem often caused by insufficient fiber in the diet. Whole grains or bran in bread and breakfast cereals and plenty of vegetables and fruits can help treat and prevent constipation. Left untreated, it may lead to other problems, such as hemorrhoids and diverticular disease—the formation of diverticulae, or pouches, in the large intestine, which can become infected and inflamed and possibly require hospital admission.

Celiac disease
A disorder known as celiac disease is caused by intolerance to gluten, a protein found in wheat, rye, and to a lesser extent, other cereal grains. Celiac disease tends to run in families. In those who suffer from it, gluten damages the walls of the intestines and prevents the absorption of various nutrients, leading to weight loss, anemia, excessive gas, and chronic diarrhea. Avoiding gluten by substituting gluten-free bread and pasta, rice, corn, potatoes, and beans for the troublesome cereal products can restore normal function of the intestines and enable a celiac sufferer to lead a normal life.

Migraines
Certain foods, including chocolate, cheese, and coffee, can trigger a migraine in susceptible individuals. Migraine is characterized by severe pain on one side of the head, sometimes accompanied by nausea, vomiting, and visual disturbances. Avoiding culprit foods can help prevent migraine attacks.

DISORDERS THAT RESPOND TO DIETARY CHANGES

From diabetes to constipation, many conditions are affected by the foods you eat and respond well to a change in diet. On the other hand, certain genetic disorders will show little or no response to diet, although sometimes the side effects and symptoms of these disorders can be relieved through dietary changes.

Diet-unresponsive	Seemingly diet-unresponsive	Partly diet-responsive	Wholly diet-responsive
conditions, such as congenital blindness or deafness,.tend to be predetermined at birth.	diseases, such as osteoporosis and cancer, may respond to or have the risk reduced through dietary means.	disorders, in which symptoms and risk can be reduced, include many circulatory and metabolic problems.	diseases, such as vitamin and mineral deficiencies, can be completely cured by dietary adjustments.

DIETARY FACTORS IN DISEASE

DISORDER	DIETARY FACTORS	PRACTICAL MEASURES
Obesity, diabetes, hypertension	Too many calories, especially from fat; excess calories will be stored as flab.	Fill up on starchy foods, not fats, and eat plenty of fruits and vegetables.
Obesity, some cancers, heart disease	Too much fat, especially saturated fat, raises cholesterol levels.	Use low-fat products and steam, boil, stir-fry, or bake foods instead of frying.
Constipation, diverticular disease, heart disease, some cancers	Inadequate fiber intake interferes with digestion and raises cholesterol levels.	Eat whole-grain breads and pasta, brown rice, and plenty of fruits and vegetables.
Anemia	Inadequate iron intake damages oxygen-carrying capacity of blood.	Eat meat, fish, iron-enriched cereals, legumes, vitamin C- and zinc-rich foods.
Osteoporosis	Inadequate intake of calcium, magnesium, and vitamin D weakens bones.	Eat low-fat dairy products, leafy green vegetables, sesame seeds, legumes, and calcium-fortified products.
Hypertension	Excess sodium intake and inadequate amounts of calcium, magnesium, and potassium can raise blood pressure.	Eat whole-grain cereals, bananas, and low-fat dairy products. Cut back on salt intake.
Many cancers	Antioxidants help fight free radicals, which can cause cancer.	Eat a wide variety of fruits and vegetables.

Eczema

Another nutrition-responsive disease that frequently affects young children who have a family history of asthma and hay fever is eczema. It is characterized by redness of the skin, itching, and blistering. Allergies to such foods as milk and eggs commonly spark eczema, so a change in diet can sometimes improve the condition quickly.

DIET AND OBESITY

Obesity is the most common nutritional disorder in this country, and it is on the increase. Although many people blame their weight on a sluggish metabolism or a hormone imbalance, the major cause is an excess intake of energy (calories in food) coupled with an inactive lifestyle. Obesity can rapidly respond to a change in diet and an increase in physical activity. Dietary habits are hard to shift, as they are often passed from generation to generation, but once modified they can become part of a healthier lifestyle. Current nutritional guidelines suggest increasing your intake of complex carbohydrates (starches) by eating more foods such as potatoes, pasta, beans, rice, bread, and cereals and reducing the amount of fat in your diet. Obesity will definitely respond to these simple approaches and to regular exercise. By avoiding obesity you can greatly reduce your risk of developing late-onset diabetes in middle age.

DIABETES

Late-onset diabetes, otherwise known as non-insulin-dependent diabetes mellitus (NIDDM), tends to occur in people who are obese. This is because enlarged fat cells interfere with the body's normal metabolic processes. If you already suffer from diabetes, diet plays an important part in controlling it. A low-fat, high-complex- carbohydrate diet with plenty of fresh fruits and vegetables will ensure that blood glucose levels are kept under control. This regimen can also help you maintain a stable weight and reduce the risk of cardiovascular problems, which are common in diabetics.

CARDIOVASCULAR PROBLEMS

There is unanimous agreement among doctors and scientists that the risk of coronary artery disease can be greatly reduced by keeping weight stable at its optimum level and blood cholesterol low.

High levels of blood cholesterol tend to run in families, but a diet low in saturated fats will reduce cholesterol. In some cases, appropriate drug treatment may also be

THE NATION'S HEALTH

In recent years many governments have set targets to reduce several widespread disorders and improve the health of their populations through nutrition education. Some of the conditions under special scrutiny include:

▶ *Hypertension*
▶ *Heart disease*
▶ *Cancer*
▶ *Obesity*
▶ *Poor growth in children of low-income families*
▶ *Susceptibility to infection in low-income populations*

DEFICIENCY DISEASES

Some of the more serious, but fortunately rarer, deficiency diseases are:

▶ *Beriberi, a degenerative nerve disorder, caused by a lack of vitamin B₁ (thiamine)*

▶ *Pellagra, characterized by dermatitis, diarrhea, and dementia, which results from a lack of vitamin B₃ (niacin)*

▶ *Rickets (in children) and osteomalacia (in adults), in which bones remain too soft and become distorted as a result of insufficient vitamin D.*

▶ *Scurvy, characterized by spongy gums, loosened teeth, and internal bleeding, which results from a severe lack of vitamin C (see page 17).*

necessary. Simple ways to reduce saturated fat intake are to replace whole-milk products with low-fat or nonfat varieties and eat meat less often.

Key risk factors for stroke are high blood pressure, arteriosclerosis, heart disease, and diabetes. Hypertension, or high blood pressure, runs in families, but blood pressure also tends to rise with age, smoking, and excessive use of alcohol. A diet low in salt and high in potassium—from dried fruits, bananas, citrus fruits, avocados, legumes, and whole grains—can help control blood pressure and decrease the risk of stroke.

CANCER

Cancer is increasingly being linked to diet. Some experts believe that as many as one in three cancers may be diet related. Because cancer is a multistage disease, however, it is difficult to determine precisely what role diet plays. Evidence suggests that diets high in fruits and vegetables, low in fat, and based predominantly on starchy foods lessen the likelihood of developing cancer.

OSTEOPOROSIS

Loss of bone density, or osteoporosis, resulting in an increased risk of fractures, affects many elderly women in this country. Although there is a genetic component, a high calcium intake, especially during the

teenage and young adult years, coupled with regular exercise, is now thought to be the best way of preventing the disease.

SIGNS OF DEFICIENCY

A very poor diet can lead to various vitamin and mineral deficiencies that will improve only when foods rich in the deficient nutrients are eaten or supplements that contain them are taken. Today severe nutritional diseases (such as those described in the far left column) are rare in the Western world, but an insufficient amount over time of any vitamins and minerals for which dietary allowances have been established can lead to unpleasant and even health-threatening symptoms.

A common problem is anemia, characterized by constant fatigue and weakness. It is caused most often by lack of iron but sometimes vitamin B₁₂ and/or folic acid. Meat, especially liver, is a fine source of all the above; legumes, green leafy vegetables, and fortified cereals contain iron and folic acid.

Without sufficient vitamin D, either from exposure to sunlight or foods rich in the vitamin—for example, cod-liver oil and eggs—the bones do not properly absorb calcium and phosphorous. Today milk and milk products are fortified with vitamin D to prevent this problem, but a person who can't tolerate milk or get outdoors is susceptible.

Too little vitamin A can lead to very dry skin and eyes, night blindness, and increased susceptibility to infection; a child's growth may be stunted. All orange and yellow fruits and vegetables are rich sources.

A severe lack of Vitamin B₂, found in animal foods and fortified cereals, is evidenced by vision problems and mouth sores. Depression, confusion, and unexplained weight loss can result from deprivation of Vitamin B₆. It is plentiful in so many foods, however, that such deficiency is rare.

The body depends on vitamin K for proper clotting of the blood. Too little of this nutrient can result in excessive bleeding and easy bruising. Cruciferous and leafy green vegetables, milk, and liver are good sources.

Insufficient amounts of potassium and/or magnesium can lead to muscle weakness and cardiac arrhythmia. Potassium is also a factor in hypertension (see above).

Zinc deficiency can cause lowered immune function, slow healing of wounds, and in children, stunted growth. Meat, seafood, and fortified cereals are good providers of zinc.

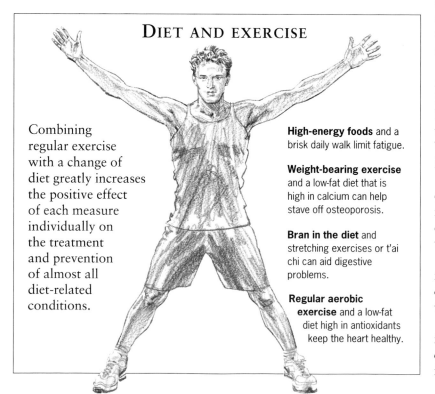

DIET AND EXERCISE

Combining regular exercise with a change of diet greatly increases the positive effect of each measure individually on the treatment and prevention of almost all diet-related conditions.

High-energy foods and a brisk daily walk limit fatigue.

Weight-bearing exercise and a low-fat diet that is high in calcium can help stave off osteoporosis.

Bran in the diet and stretching exercises or t'ai chi can aid digestive problems.

Regular aerobic exercise and a low-fat diet high in antioxidants keep the heart healthy.

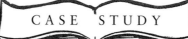
A Migraine Sufferer

Migraine can often be triggered by a food intolerance, in which the body reacts abnormally to a food—common offenders being chocolate, caffeine, cheese, citrus fruits, and red wine. If the food in question is eaten daily or if the reaction is delayed, the connection between food and symptoms may not be obvious.

Ian is a 35-year-old father of three and a part-time student. He is married to Sarah, who does not sympathize with his frequent migraine attacks or the difficulty he has concentrating while studying. Their marriage has been shaky for several years, and Ian is seeing a counselor for stress. He has had migraines for about eight years, and both the counselor and Ian's doctor tell him they are stress related. Ian disagrees. He is certain that when the migraine attacks first began he was not under stress but going through a very happy period in his life. Although his diet is generally good, he has decided to consult a nutritionist (see page 92) because he is worried about continuing the drugs he takes for the migraines.

WHAT SHOULD IAN DO?

Ian's nutritionist recognizes that Ian is prone to allergies. He had eczema when he was a baby and has suffered on and off with hay fever. She gives Ian a diagnostic diet to follow, having him avoid some of the most common problem foods for allergy sufferers, including milk, gluten, and foods containing caffeine. Ian will follow this diet for two weeks and then, in a carefully controlled procedure, reintroduce these foods one at a time. After his problem foods have been identified, Ian has to avoid them entirely for at least six months. He must also follow advice that will help him improve his digestion and the function of his intestines in order to become more resistant to allergies.

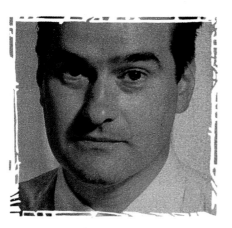

STRESS
Allergic reactions are more likely to occur when you are under stress.

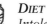

DIET
Intolerances to such foods as wheat and milk are common and can cause a variety of problems.

HEALTH
Inhaled chemicals and fumes can be very stressful to your immune system, which helps to protect you from allergies.

Action Plan

DIET
While waiting for the diagnosis, eat substitute foods like special no-gluten breads and soy milk or goat's milk. Ask the nutritionist about taking supplements.

STRESS
Find out about attending meditation classes. Seek advice on relaxation techniques.

HEALTH
Avoid using aerosols, such as hairspray, perfume, deodorants, spray polishes, and artificially perfumed air fresheners.

HOW THINGS TURNED OUT FOR IAN

Ian discovered that dairy products were the culprits. From the moment he started the diagnostic diet, he had no migraines at all, but symptoms began a few hours after he drank tea with milk. Two years later Ian is still migraine free and no longer develops a fuzzy-headed feeling when studying. This improvement has helped him pass all his exams. Best of all, Ian's marriage has improved with his better state of health, and he feels in control of his life again.

THE IMMUNE SYSTEM

A balanced diet that contains all the essential nutrients is the most important factor for proper functioning of the cells and tissues that constitute the immune system.

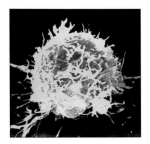

IMMUNE CELLS
White blood cells are essential in the fight against disease and infection. A special white blood cell called a memory cell (illustrated above) recognizes and destroys infectious microorganisms when they appear. This is how people develop immunity to diseases like mumps.

The air, food, and water essential for life all contain foreign substances and microorganisms such as bacteria and viruses. Many of these substances are harmless, but others can quickly interfere with the body's functions and cause infections and diseases. The skin, lungs, and digestive system are all lined with protective membranes that prevent foreign substances from entering the body. If some do penetrate these barriers, however, it is the role of the immune cells, or white blood cells, to remove these foreign substances before they get the chance to do harm.

The immune system doesn't consist only of the white blood cells. Stomach acid kills bacteria and parasites ingested with your food. Your intestines contain friendly bacteria that destroy harmful microorganisms that get past the stomach. Your liver is vital to breaking down poisonous chemicals from food, air, and water, as well as creating bile, which is vital to the breakdown of fats in your digestive system.

FOODS AND IMMUNITY
Several conditions, including malabsorption problems and severe malnutrition, can damage the immune system, thus increasing the risk of life-threatening infections. A healthy diet can redress any imbalances and boost the immune system considerably.

Vitamins
The immune system needs all of the known vitamins (13) to function properly. Researchers believe that more vitamins probably exist than have been identified, which is the reason eating a broad range of foods is advised.

Certain vitamins do seem to play a more significant role than others in immune function, however. Vitamin A is needed for the immune cells to develop properly. Together with other antioxidants, vitamins C and E, it destroys the excess free radicals produced by immune cells when they attack bacteria and viruses (see chapter 3). Further, vitamin E is an antioxidant that protects cell membranes from free radical attack. Even when

THE IMMUNE RESPONSE

White blood cells called phagocytes are attracted to infection sites, where they destroy bacteria, immobilize virus particles, and help repair damaged cells. The remains of the alien cell, left behind by the effect of the lysosomes in the white blood cell, are then expelled from the body.

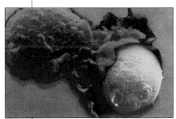

PHAGOCYTOSIS
A white blood cell is in the process of engulfing an alien particle.

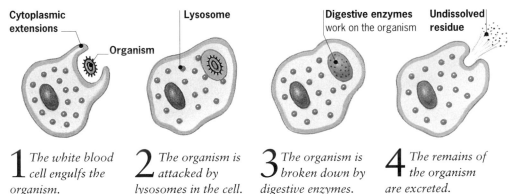

Cytoplasmic extensions — **Organism**

Lysosome

Digestive enzymes work on the organism

Undissolved residue

1 *The white blood cell engulfs the organism.*

2 *The organism is attacked by lysosomes in the cell.*

3 *The organism is broken down by digestive enzymes.*

4 *The remains of the organism are excreted.*

vitamins do not have a specific role to play in immune function, deficiencies will increase susceptibility to infection by compromising important functions in the body.

When the Nobel laureate Linus Pauling claimed in 1970 that large doses of vitamin C reduced the likelihood of contracting colds, many people began to take megadoses of it. Since then, clinical trials have failed to prove this claim; the body does need this vitamin daily, but not in megadoses.

Minerals

Many minerals are required for the immune system to respond correctly. The most important one is iron, which is required to form certain immune cells. Iron deficiency not only can impair this process but also can lessen the capacity of immune cells to kill bacteria. On a vegetarian diet it is more difficult to obtain sufficient iron because iron is less easily absorbed from plant foods. Combining iron-rich foods with those high in vitamin C can improve absorption.

Zinc deficiency can also lead to impaired immune function. Also, a zinc-deficient diet during pregnancy delays normal development of the immune system in the fetus.

AN OVEREAGER IMMUNE SYSTEM

All people who suffer from food allergies are actually feeling the effects of massive attacks from their own immune systems. Although it is essential for immune cells to respond quickly to outside invaders, in these cases the immune system overreacts and starts attacking the body's own cells. The immune system is treating a food particle like a germ and releasing antibodies that activate inflammatory substances and result in a range of symptoms. Individuals who suffer from such attacks need to pinpoint the problem food and remove it from the diet.

Rheumatoid arthritis, osteoarthritis, and lupus are examples of autoimmune diseases. Sometimes diet can be used to modulate the immune system and decrease symptoms. Many arthritis sufferers respond well, for example, to a decrease in high-fat meats and any foods that seem to provoke a flare-up.

Oily fish and fish oil supplements, which contain omega-3 fatty acids, may in many cases stimulate some of the overactive immune cells to produce less inflammatory agents in the joints. This in turn can decrease the inflammation and relieve pain.

VITAMIN C MEGADOSES

Very high doses of vitamin C (5,000 mg or more per day) can cause diarrhea, urinary tract irritation, and kidney stones. In susceptible people, supplements of vitamin C above 200 mg per day may cause dangerous excesses of iron in the body because this vitamin increases iron absorption.

Evening primrose oil has similar effects and may be useful for anyone who does not eat fish. These two supplements must never be used, however, without the supervision of a doctor; they can be dangerous in large doses.

Lupus, a chronic autoimmune disease characterized by debilitating fatigue, joint pain, skin rashes, and dry mouth, can be worsened by sun exposure and certain foods. Foods that worsen symptoms in some lupus sufferers are alfafa and possibly other legumes, mushrooms, and smoked foods. Those who are sensitive to the sun should avoid celery, parsley, lemons, limes, and parsnips, all of which heighten photosensitivity. Many lupus patients note an improvement after they decrease consumption of fatty animal foods, such as meat, whole milk, and cheese.

Other factors that affect immunity

Don't forget that stress can weaken your immune system. People who lead stressful lives often neglect their diet, drink too much coffee and alcohol, and may not get the full complement of nutrients that their body needs. They are also more likely to suffer from recurrent infections. It is important to find time to relax as often as possible. Regular physical activity also reduces stress and promotes good health.

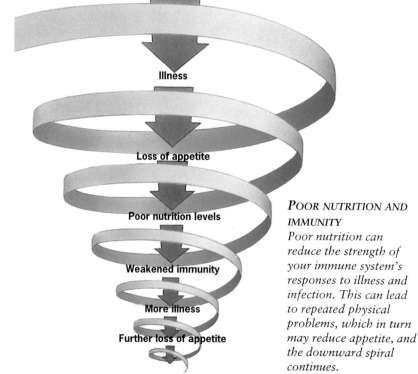

Illness

Loss of appetite

Poor nutrition levels

Weakened immunity

More illness

Further loss of appetite

POOR NUTRITION AND IMMUNITY
Poor nutrition can reduce the strength of your immune system's responses to illness and infection. This can lead to repeated physical problems, which in turn may reduce appetite, and the downward spiral continues.

Immune System

Like any function of the body, the immune system needs adequate nutrients to keep it working at its best; a deficiency in any one can make the body more susceptible to infection. Eating all the right foods can definitely boost the immune system.

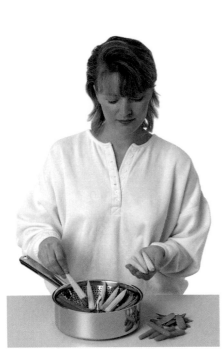

COOKING TO PRESERVE VITAMINS
Lightly cooking vegetables by steaming, stir-frying, or boiling in as little water as possible will help preserve their vitamins.

Several nutrients are important to the proper functioning of the immune system. Among them are the antioxidant vitamins, A, C, and E. These counteract the effects of free radicals, which can damage cells and disrupt the body's defenses.

Iron and zinc have major roles in keeping the immune system strong. Zinc supports numerous bodily functions, particularly the activity of many enzymes, so even a small deficiency can have an impact. People who are anemic because of insufficient iron, B_{12} and/or zinc are more prone to illness, and any injuries they incur will be slow to heal.

The B vitamins—folate, B_6, and B_{12}—are also involved in supporting the immune system. And there is a great deal of evidence that garlic has antiviral, antifungal, and antibacterial properties that help both to prevent and to fight infection.

The importance of fiber
Your liver fights foreign bodies such as bacteria and breaks them down into waste products. Fiber-rich foods like vegetables, fruits, whole grains, and legumes are needed to hasten the emptying of your bowels and prevent your intestines from reabsorbing your liver's waste products.

FOODS TO HELP THE IMMUNE SYSTEM

Homemade soups are simple to make and provide an easy way to get your daily servings of vegetables. To prepare lentil soup, sauté some chopped onion and garlic. Add 1 pound of lentils, a few chopped tomatoes, and water and bring to a boil. Simmer for an hour or until thick; season to taste.

It makes good sense to add to your soups the water in which you have cooked vegetables for a main course; it contains water-soluble vitamins.

Another way to boost your immune system is with homemade juices. Good combinations include broccoli and apple; tomato, carrot, and lemon; apple and pear. Drink juice immediately because vitamin C breaks down on exposure to air.

FRESH JUICE
With a juice extractor you can make your own vitamin-rich fruit and vegetable juices.

HOMEMADE SOUP
Like homemade juices, homemade soups are a convenient way to add more fiber and vitamins to your diet. In addition to lentil soup (far left), other variations you can try are leek and potato (top) and broccoli and cauliflower (bottom). All are nourishing, especially when served with a swirl of yogurt or a sprinkling of grated low-fat cheese.

CANCER

It is estimated that at least one-third of cancerous malignancies are related to diet. Many of these could probably be prevented with dietary changes.

When body cells become disturbed, they may start to divide erratically and invade surrounding tissues. Factors that can disturb cells include radiation, viruses, certain chemicals in the environment, and tobacco smoking. Cancer is a multistage process, with various cancer-causing agents, or carcinogens, promoting chaotic cell division, and other substances, or anticarcinogens, preventing it.

FOODS THAT CAN CAUSE CANCER

It is well established that diet plays a role in the development of some cancers. Cancers that have been linked to diet include those of the mouth and throat, stomach, large intestine, pancreas, liver, gallbladder, lung, breast, uterus, ovaries, and prostate.

Food contains various carcinogens. Both carcinogens and anticarcinogens may occur in the same food. For example, fruits and vegetables may contain naturally occurring carcinogens or the residues of pesticides, but they also contain various antioxidants that can protect you.

Many substances that occur naturally in foods have been shown to cause cancer in laboratory animals. These originate mostly in plants, in particular, certain herbs and spices. However, your risk of developing cancer from eating these plant foods is minimal.

Molds

Molds, such as those sometimes found on peanuts, can contain potent cancer-causing chemicals called aflatoxins. A similar mold called ochratoxin grows on cereals stored under damp conditions. These molds occur mostly in the tropics; in North America food storage is generally well controlled.

FACTORS THAT MAY CONTRIBUTE TO CANCER

▶ *A high risk for certain cancers is inherited.*

▶ *Substances like asbestos and chemicals from car exhaust fumes are known carcinogens.*

▶ *Smoking is the major cause of lung cancer.*

▶ *Certain viruses can cause cancer; an example is human papilloma virus in cervical cancer.*

▶ *Ultraviolet light from sun causes skin cancer.*

▶ *Radiation increases the risk of certain cancers.*

HOW CANCER DEVELOPS

A carcinogen is a substance that causes body cells to change. Cells that develop abnormally after exposure to a carcinogen are described as cancerous. Initially this disruption spreads from cell to cell, but the spread can also move from one part of the body to another.

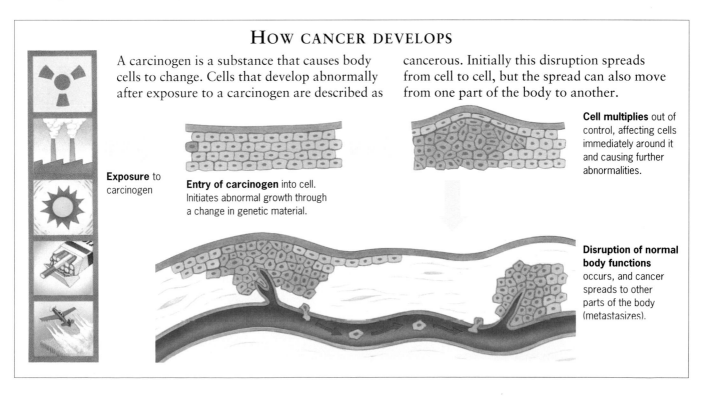

Exposure to carcinogen

Entry of carcinogen into cell. Initiates abnormal growth through a change in genetic material.

Cell multiplies out of control, affecting cells immediately around it and causing further abnormalities.

Disruption of normal body functions occurs, and cancer spreads to other parts of the body (metastasizes).

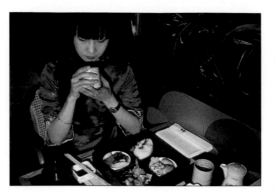

RAW FISH
The Japanese diet, which includes large quantities of raw fish and soy products, seems to be beneficial in preventing certain cancers. Japan's overall rate of cancer is much lower than that in Western countries.

Bad habits

A high alcohol intake has been linked to cancers of the mouth, throat, and liver, particularly in people who also smoke. It seems that the combined effects of alcohol and smoking greatly increase the risk of these cancers. Coffee consumption, if moderate, has not been linked to cancer, although very high intakes may increase the risk.

Pollution and foods

Industrial pollutants released into the atmosphere can contaminate food when deposited on crops. Tobacco smoke also contains high levels of harmful compounds. And the charred residue on meat that has been barbecued has been implicated in cancer of the esophagus and stomach.

Residues from chemical pesticides and fertilizers are a great cause for concern. Traces of such chemicals have found their way into fruits, vegetables, fish, and milk. Lindane, found in milk, is one such chemical that has been linked to breast cancer in women, although the evidence is not yet conclusive.

Additives

Other substances suspected of causing cancer are food additives. In North America these are vigorously tested before they are permitted for use in foods. In fact, more is known about the potential hazards of food additives than about the risks posed by naturally occurring substances in food. Additives are present in minute amounts in our diet and are highly unlikely to contribute to cancer. Indeed, some experimental evidence shows that various synthetic antioxidants added to some margarines and fat-containing foods to prevent the fat from going rancid can inhibit the formation of cancer.

Fats and cancer

A diet high in fat, especially animal fat, may cause the body to produce an excess of hormones that help tumors to grow; promote bile secretion, which may stimulate tumor growth; or change cell structure and enable cancer to form. Some fats are more closely linked to cancer development than others.

A diet that is too high in calories, particularly in the form of fat, can lead to obesity. Cancers of the uterus, gallbladder, kidney, stomach, colon, and breast are significantly higher in obese people (those who are 20 percent over their ideal weight). Obesity alters various protective mechanisms in the body, such as immune function and hormone levels. These changes appear to create favorable conditions for cancers to develop.

Meats

The high temperatures used to fry, broil, or grill meat create potential cancer-causing substances. The longer meat (also poultry and fish) is cooked, the more these compounds are produced; roasting, braising, and poaching produce few or none.

The fat that drips onto hot coals, stones, or coils when meat is grilled can also produce potential carcinogens. Smoke deposits these chemicals on the food.

FOODS THAT PROTECT AGAINST CANCER

Various foods are believed to help protect against cancer, although no food can be claimed as a cure for it.

The protective role of fiber

Colon cancer has been linked to a high-fat, low-fiber diet. Fiber encourages the growth of friendly bacteria in the large intestine and ensures that the gut functions properly. It also binds excess bile and other harmful by-products of digestion, thus preventing them from adhering to the bowel wall.

Some starches from foods like potatoes and pasta resist digestion in the small intestine but can be fermented by friendly bacteria in the large bowel. Certain fatty acids produced by the bacteria during this process may protect the bowel wall against carcinogens. It is

THE RISK OF CANCER THROUGH FOODS

Some foods that are considered healthful can actually pose a cancer risk, depending on how they are packaged, preserved, or cooked. For example, barbecuing meat can produce substances that are considered carcinogenic.

Pesticides can contaminate dairy products.

Improper storage can lead to the growth of hazardous molds.

Carcinogens can form in meat that is charred during cooking.

Breast Cancer Risk

Cross-cultural studies suggest that diet may play a far more significant part in health and the development of breast cancer than was generally assumed. Many lives may be saved if women understand and implement appropriate changes to their diet.

Two dietary aspects have been identified with the risk of developing breast cancer: being overweight and not eating enough vegetables and fruits. Too much fat and too little fiber in the diet may also be factors, but long-term studies have, so far, proved otherwise. In countries like Japan, however, where dietary intake of animal fat is low, there is a lower incidence of breast cancer. Some experts still suspect that fat is a culprit.

A known risk factor for breast cancer in postmenopausal women is excessive weight gain around the abdomen, breasts, shoulders, and nape of the neck.

Fruits and vegetables contain large amounts of the antioxidant vitamins, A, C, and E. These protect the body from tissue damage caused by oxidation and also appear to prevent the development of cancerous cells.

Antioxidant sources

Rich sources of vitamin A include eggs, liver, milk and milk products, green leafy vegetables, tomatoes, and orange and yellow vegetables and fruits like carrots and apricots. Vitamin C is plentiful in citrus fruits, berries, melons, potatoes, peppers, and cabbage, and vitamin E in vegetable oils, avocados, and nuts of all kinds.

BREAST CANCER AROUND THE WORLD
Incidences of breast cancer in North America and northern Europe (red) are among the highest in the world, with Japan and Hong Kong (blue), among the lowest. All the regions colored yellow have relatively low rates. A trend is emerging that as poorer countries become more affluent, or as Western habits and diets are adopted by those countries, rates of breast cancer increase.

A DIET PLAN TO REDUCE THE RISK

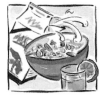

BREAKFAST
Pour nonfat or low-fat milk on your cereal and sprinkle a handful of nuts and seeds on top, such as sunflower or pumpkin seeds. Eat a piece of fresh fruit or have a glass of fruit juice with no added sugar.

LUNCH
If you have a sandwich for lunch, choose a whole-grain bread and a filling that is low in animal fat, such as chicken, a bean or nut spread, canned fish, or low-fat cheese. Include a piece of fruit as well.

EVENING MEAL
Serve small quantities of meat with the main course and try to have an alternative to meat, such as fish, cheese, eggs, or beans, three or four times a week. Include at least two vegetables in the meal—one green and one root (potatoes or carrots, for example). Choose sorbet or low-fat yogurt for dessert. If you are trying to lose weight, have dessert only occasionally .

REDUCING THE RISK

▶ *Reduce your intake of saturated animal fats found in whole-milk dairy foods and fatty meats.*
▶ *Maintain your ideal weight.*
▶ *Eat foods rich in vitamin E, such as pumpkin and sesame seeds, nuts, whole grains, fortified cereals, leafy greens, and vegetable oils.*
▶ *Eat less animal protein or adopt a balanced vegetarian diet.*
▶ *Reduce your intake of salt, refined sugar, alcohol, and caffeinated drinks.*
▶ *Increase your intake of fresh vegetables and fruit.*
▶ *Eat more soy products, such as soy milk, tofu, and tempeh—all good sources of phytoestrogen (see page 40).*
▶ *Eat cruciferous vegetables like broccoli and cabbage—excellent sources of indoles (see page 40).*

Folic acid and cervical cancer

Cervical cancer is caused by the human papilloma virus, which is activated in the body under certain conditions. It is thought that activation of the virus is more likely in the absence of folic acid (folate). Adequate folic acid is therefore important protection against cervical cancer. Rich sources include spinach and other dark leafy greens, nuts, cruciferous vegetables, liver, fortified cereals, and dried legumes. Frequent use of medications such as aspirin may deplete folic acid in your body, so if you are on medication, eat folic-acid-rich foods.

not just fiber and digestion-resistant starch that are thought to protect against bowel cancer but also the antioxidant nutrients and other substances in fruits and vegetables.

Vitamin C and cancer

Stomach cancer is prevalent in countries like Japan, where a lot of smoked, salted, and pickled foods are consumed. In addition to their high salt content, these foods often contain preservative nitrites and nitrates, which produce carcinogens called nitrosamines, known to cause cancer in laboratory animals. (Some vegetables, such as celery, are naturally high in nitrates.) Although the amounts people ingest from food are low and regarded as being within safe limits, it is worth cutting down on preserved meats and smoked fish and eating more fruits and vegetables that contain vitamin C, which prevents the formation of nitrosamines both in food and in the stomach.

Low levels of vitamin C in the blood have been linked to abnormal cervical smears in women who smoke. Because smoking depletes vitamin C rapidly in the body, smokers should take at least double the recommended daily intake, or 120 mg. Two large oranges will provide this amount. Better still, give up smoking. This habit is known to cause lung cancer and is also associated with cancer of the mouth, throat, pancreas, and bladder.

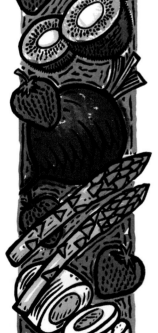

ANTICANCER FOODS

Some foods contain specific compounds that may help protect cells against the formation and spread of cancer.

CANCER	SUGGESTED FOODS
General	Fruits and vegetables (vitamin C, bioflavonoids), seafood, poultry, whole grains (selenium), garlic, onions (sulfur compounds), chickpeas, lima beans (protease inhibitors), eggs (vitamin E)
Breast	Broccoli, cabbage, soybeans, tofu, (indoles and phytoestrogen)
Lung	Fruits and vegetables (vitamin C)
Stomach	Fewer smoked, pickled, salted foods; more fruits and vegetables
Cervical	Liver, legumes, avocados (folate)

DIETARY RECOMMENDATIONS FOR PREVENTING CANCER

International experts in nutrition agree that a high intake of fruits and vegetables greatly reduces the risk of cancer, probably because they conatain an abundance of the antioxidant vitamins C, E, and beta carotene (precursor to vitamin A), plus other phytochemicals, the roles of which have yet to be determined.

The antioxidant mineral selenium offers the same protection. Selenium is abundant in seafood, poultry, lean meats, whole grains, and brazil nuts. Antioxidant nutrients are thought to work by neutralizing free radicals (see page 50), which, left unchecked, can interfere with a cell's genetic material and initiate cancer.

Some B vitamins may also play protective roles. Riboflavin (vitamin B_2), pyridoxine (vitamin B_6), and folic acid are all involved in neutralizing potential carcinogens.

Other beneficial substances

There are many more substances in fruits and vegetables, including the carotenoids lutein and lycopene in kale, spinach, and tomatoes, which can interact with each other to help prevent cancer.

Other plant chemicals known as indoles, found in broccoli, kale, cabbage, and other cruciferous vegetables, have been shown to interfere with the action of the female hormone estrogen, rendering it less potent in breast tumors that rely on estrogen for growth. Soybeans and other soy products like tofu contain plant hormones known as phytoestrogens, which have a similar effect.

Sulphur compounds in garlic and onions, other compounds in cruciferous vegetables (such as isothiocyanates and phenols), and bioflavonoids, which are present in most fruits and vegetables, have been shown to be important in inhibiting cancer. Protease inhibitors, found in soybeans, chickpeas, other legumes, and potatoes, are thought to inhibit the enzymes that help tumors grow.

OBESITY

Despite advice from health experts about the importance of avoiding obesity, it appears to be increasing. Being overweight is the most prevalent diet-related health problem in America.

About one-third of adult Americans are seriously overweight, or obese, defined as being 20 percent above the ideal weight for height, body type, and age. The costs of obesity are enormous in terms of decreased health and longevity.

HEALTH PROBLEMS CAUSED BY OBESITY

Apart from the self-image and social issues associated with excess weight, obesity also greatly increases the risk of premature death. Coronary artery disease is more prevalent among obese individuals; weight gain is associated with increased blood pressure and blood cholesterol levels—two major risk factors for heart disease and stroke. Obese persons are also more likely to develop osteoarthritis of weight-bearing joints, especially the back, hips, and knees. Disability from this disease is likely to restrict activities, thus leading to even more weight gain.

Overweight women have a higher risk of developing cancers of the breast, ovaries, endometrium, and cervix. These are cancers that depend on hormones, and they are associated particularly with high levels of the hormone estrogen, which is produced in excess in fat women and stored in fat cells. Hormonal imbalances in obese women also lead frequently to menstrual problems. Obese men have an increased risk of cancers of the large intestine and prostate. Obese individuals, in general, are also more likely to develop diabetes, gallstones, and gout.

The distribution of body fat in an obese person is also important. Storing fat within the abdomen is more dangerous than storing it around the hips. Fat cells in the abdomen are much more active than those found under the skin around the hips and thighs. They can release fats and cholesterol into the bloodstream, increasing the risk of many of the diseases mentioned above.

MAINTAINING HEALTHY WEIGHT

Many people embark on extreme weight-reducing diets, hoping for instant results. Unfortunately, crash diets, often consisting of low-calorie meal-replacement drinks or fasting, rarely work. The initial success is quickly replaced by disappointment as the lost weight returns with normal eating.

Many slimmers embark on a series of diets, with each period of weight loss quickly followed by one of weight gain. This is known as the yo-yo effect. Such people usually find it more difficult to lose weight each time they try because the weight they gain

WHY PEOPLE GET FAT

Many factors contribute to obesity. They vary from person to person and include overeating, a sedentary lifestyle, genetic influences, hormonal imbalances, psychological problems, slow metabolic rate, and lack of knowledge about healthy eating.

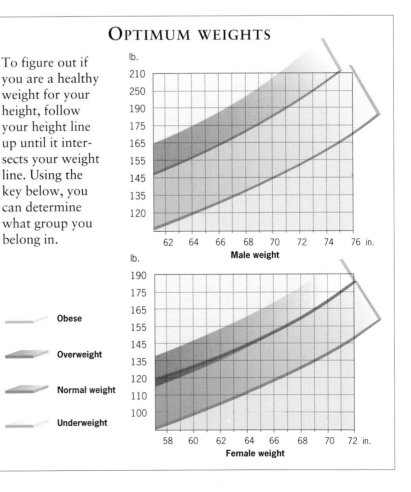

OPTIMUM WEIGHTS

To figure out if you are a healthy weight for your height, follow your height line up until it intersects your weight line. Using the key below, you can determine what group you belong in.

Obese
Overweight
Normal weight
Underweight

41

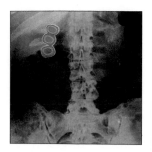

PREVENTING GALLSTONES
The most common cause of gallstones (the blue spheres to the left of the spinal column, above) is obesity. Several studies have shown that a vegetarian diet protects against the formation of gallstones. It is not known whether this is due to the absence of animal proteins and fats or the naturally higher fiber content of the vegetarian menu. It is known that plant proteins, as found in soybeans and other legumes, discourage the formation of gallstones. It may be also that the lecithin content of plant proteins helps break down bile.

between each diet is often greater than the weight they lost. Rapidly fluctuating weight has been found to increase the risk of cardiovascular disease.

Reducing weight

A weight-reducing diet should start with reducing calories from fat, which will automatically reduce total calorie intake. Fat provides twice as many calories (9 per gram) as a similar weight of protein or carbohydrate (4 calories per gram). Cutting down on whole-milk dairy products and replacing these with nonfat or low-fat ver-

SUBSTITUTE FOODS

Whenever possible, replace high-fat foods with low-fat or nonfat versions. Replacing alcohol with fruit juice not only reduces calories (4 per gram versus 7) but also improves nutrition.

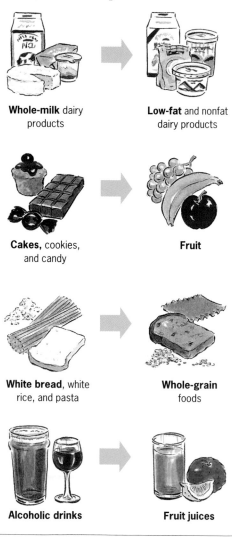

Whole-milk dairy products → **Low-fat** and nonfat dairy products

Cakes, cookies, and candy → **Fruit**

White bread, white rice, and pasta → **Whole-grain** foods

Alcoholic drinks → **Fruit juices**

sions is one way to reduce fat intake. Another is to eat less meat and fried foods .

The main bulk of the diet should come from complex carbohydrates and at least five to seven servings of fruit and vegetables each day, with moderate amounts of lean meat, skinless poultry, and fish Use alcohol in moderation—no more than one or two drinks a day. Reserve cakes, pastries, and cookies for an occasional treat.

DIABETES

Non-insulin-dependent diabetes mellitus (NIDDM) is more common in the obese, especially those over age 50. It is not known why obese people develop diabetes, but it seems that their body tissues become increasingly resistant to insulin, the hormone that enables body tissues to clear glucose from the blood and thus maintain constant blood sugar levels. As people grow older and gain weight, their resistance to insulin increases. Losing weight reverses this process. Physical activity can also improve the sensitivity of body tissues to insulin.

GALLSTONES

Gallstones are a common result of obesity and are two to three times more common in women than men. Obese people tend to have high levels of cholesterol in their blood and bile (secreted by the liver to break down fats). Cholesterol can crystallize in the gallbladder and lead to gallstones.

Cutting down dramatically on fat, particularly saturated fat, is the first line of defense against gallstone attacks. Some doctors recommend cutting fat to 10 to 20 percent of total daily calories. This means eliminating virtually all animal fats, which will lower cholesterol levels in the blood. Small amounts of polyunsaturated vegetable oils, such as sunflower oil, may be helpful because these help break down fats and maintain bile flow. Also, the monounsaturated fat in olive oil can lower cholesterol.

Adding more soluble fiber to the diet is also very important. Soluble fiber binds cholesterol and removes it from the body, so it makes sense to eat plenty of oat and rice bran, legumes, and fruits like apples.

Gallstones are linked to high consumption of refined sugar, but a moderate daily consumption of alcohol—40 ml or half a glass of wine—has been found to reduce the incidence of gallstones by half.

CARDIOVASCULAR PROBLEMS

It is estimated that more than 60 million Americans have some form of cardiovascular disease. The right diet is the single most important measure for preventing premature illness and death.

The clogging of arteries with plaque, or atherosclerosis, can start in childhood and continue throughout life with no symptoms. It begins when cholesterol in the form of low density lipoproteins (LDLs) enters through the blood vessel walls and reacts with free radicals. These are highly reactive substances formed by the body as part of its metabolism and defense against bacteria. Cholesterol is also present in the blood as high density lipoproteins (HDLs), but it is not harmful in this form. A diet high in saturated fat or a genetic predisposition can cause excess levels of LDL in the blood.

HEART AND CIRCULATORY DISEASE

Once modified by free radicals, LDL is taken up by cells inside the artery walls. Eventually some of these cells die and form fibrous plaques, or atheromas.

Atheromas

Atheromas narrow the arteries, preventing sufficient oxygen from reaching muscles when the demand increases. If the heart muscle is affected, the result is angina, characterized by a crushing pain in the chest. The pain of atheromas affecting leg muscles is known as intermittent claudication.

More seriously, if one of these plaques ruptures, it can cause a thrombus, or blood clot, to form in the artery. A clot in one of the heart arteries can lead to a heart attack. A similar clot in the brain causes a stroke.

Hypertension

High blood pressure, or hypertension, tends to increase the likelihood of stroke, heart attack, and kidney failure. Reducing salt intake may help lower mild hypertension in people who are salt sensitive and prevent blood pressure from increasing.

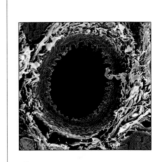

A HEALTHY ARTERY
The inner surface of a healthy artery (the purple ring in the image above) can become narrowed by fatty deposits, which prevent sufficient oxygen from reaching muscles.

Nutrition before birth
The importance of nutrition starts well before birth. Low birth weight has been associated with elevated blood pressure in adulthood, and it is well known that poorly nourished mothers have smaller babies. This was confirmed by a British study of 449 men and women, published in 1990, showing that low-weight babies had an increased risk of hypertension in adult life. Also, adequate growth and nutrition during childhood reduce the risk of developing chronic diseases later on.

RISK FACTORS FOR HEART DISEASE

Some personal factors that cannot be changed may predispose an individual to heart disease. However, the risk can be lessened by controlling those things that are within any person's control—known as the alterable risk factors.

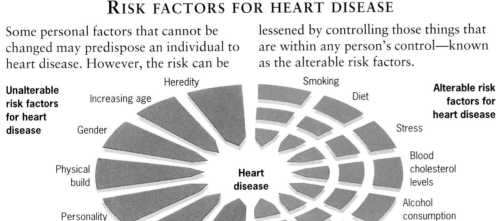

Unalterable risk factors for heart disease

Heredity
Increasing age
Gender
Physical build
Personality
Height
Diabetes

Heart disease

Alterable risk factors for heart disease

Smoking
Diet
Stress
Blood cholesterol levels
Alcohol consumption
Blood pressure
Sedentary lifestyle

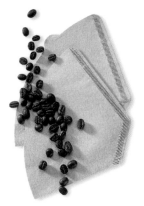

Coffee
Although caffeine makes the heart beat faster and increases blood pressure slightly, there is no evidence that caffeine in moderation can increase the risk of heart disease. However, certain substances are formed in coffee when it is boiled or made in a cafetière (French-press coffee-maker). These chemicals are associated with higher blood cholesterol levels and they seem to be removed when coffee is filtered.

Stickiness of the blood

Another important factor in the formation of a blood clot is the stickiness, or viscosity, of the blood. This is greatly increased by smoking. Viscous blood clots more easily, especially around atheromas.

DIET AND CARDIOVASCULAR PROBLEMS

Despite the fact that heart disease remains one of North America's biggest killers, there has been a dramatic decline in death rates over the past decade. This can perhaps be attributed to improved medical treatment and healthier lifestyles, including better diet.

Fats and dietary cholesterol

Japan and Mediterranean countries, which have a low consumption of saturated fats and a high one of vegetables and fruits, have low rates of heart disease. For example, the death rate from heart attacks is eight times greater in Britain than in Japan and three times greater than in Spain. Saturated fats, which increase LDLs ("bad" cholesterol) and reduce HDLs ("good" cholesterol), are the prevalent type in animal foods.

Cholesterol from foods such as eggs and shellfish seems to have a minimal effect on blood cholesterol levels in most people. However, health experts advise staying within the current recommended intake of 245 mg a day (the amount in one large egg).

Omega-3 fatty acids in oily fish, such as mackerel and sardines protect against thrombosis by making blood less viscous and therefore less likely to clot. Consuming oily fish at least once a week can add to the arsenal that protects the heart.

PROTECTION FROM PLANTS

Antioxidants, especially vitamins A, C, and E, may protect against atherosclerosis by preventing LDL cholesterol from forming plaque. Almost all fruits and vegetables contain some amounts of vitamins A and C. Vitamin E is available from wheat germ, nuts, seeds, vegetable oils, and leafy greens.

Some of the soluble fibers, namely those in pectin (present in many fruits, legumes, and some vegetables), oat and rice bran, and guar gum, are known to reduce blood cholesterol levels, which in turn lowers the risk of coronary artery disease and heart attacks.

After menopause, estrogen, which protects a woman against heart disease during her reproductive years, is greatly reduced and her risk of heart disease increases dramatically. All soy products contain high levels of plant estrogens (phytoestrogens), which seem to protect against atherosclerosis. The low rates of heart disease in Japan may be due, in part, to the high soy diet.

Alcohol

Moderate alcohol consumption, especially of red wine, may actually protect against atherosclerosis. However, drinking more than one or two glasses a day can increase blood pressure and the risk of a stroke.

DIET, HYPERTENSION, AND HEART DISEASE

Keeping blood pressure under control and preventing blood from clotting are two ways of lowering the risk of heart disease. These two goals can be accomplished in large measure by the regular inclusion of certain foods in the diet and the reduction of others.

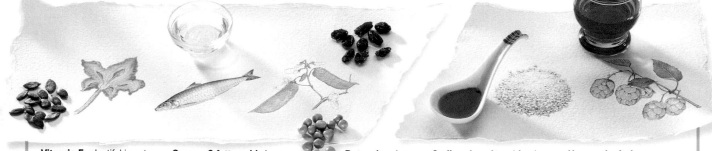

Vitamin E, plentiful in nuts and such seeds as pumpkin, inhibits blood clotting to help prevent heart attacks.

Omega-3 fatty acids in oily fish can thin blood and reduce cholesterol levels and the risk of heart disease.

Potassium in fruits and legumes balances sodium to keep blood pressure normal.

Sodium in salt and foods that are highly salted during preparation or preservation can increase hypertension.

Heavy alcohol consumption can increase blood pressure and damage the heart muscle.

Heart-Healthy Foods

Even in the presence of other risk factors, you can reduce your risk of heart disease by making dietary changes. Indeed, some people swear by a head of garlic a day, but if that is too much for you, there are other options.

Numerous studies have shown that garlic, onions, and ginger inhibit the ability of the blood to form clots and thus may reduce the risk of heart attack. Garlic also lowers cholesterol levels and high blood pressure. Exactly how much should be eaten for these effects is not certain; possibly at least 2 cloves a day are needed to lower blood pressure, 10 cloves to thin the blood.

Although garlic and onions often leave an unpleasant odor on the breath, chewing parsley or cloves can offset the effect. Also, the longer you cook garlic and onions, the less likely they are to leave an aftertaste.

Some people get indigestion from raw garlic; it can also irritate the mucous membranes. For them garlic pills may be advised, but they should consult a doctor first.

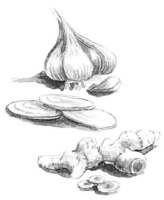

GARLIC, ONIONS, AND GINGER
Keep these three anticoagulant foods on hand in your kitchen for their healthful benefits, as well as their flavor. You can modify the amounts to suit your taste.

FAT-SAVING IDEAS

To keep the heart healthy or restore a damaged one, some doctors advise limiting fat to no more than 25 percent of daily calories, and a few have publicly advocated getting this figure down as low as 10 percent. Unquestionably, reducing levels of saturated fat is beneficial.

Using a nutritious spread on sandwiches instead of margarine or butter will give you more useful calories and less fat. Try homemade bean spread or nonfat cream cheese. If you use mayonnaise, choose a nonfat or reduced-fat version.

If you cannot bear the idea of low-fat foods, gradually add less and less of the high-fat foods you adore to each meal. Each week replace one fatty item with a low-fat substitute. If you do a little at a time, you soon won't notice the changes.

When sautéing foods, use a nonstick pan and just a little oil. You can also use the technique of "sweating," cooking onions and garlic in a little broth. Avoid frying foods. Experiment with grilling,

poaching, steaming, and baking to help cut fat out of your diet.

Sauces can easily be made creamy by using low-fat yogurt instead of cream. To make puréed soups creamy, add a couple of potatoes to them. Puréed soups in general are a good addition to a heart-healthy menu. Simply sauté some garlic and onion in a little oil, then add

your choice of vegetables, such as carrots, pumpkin, turnips, and potatoes, and nonfat or low-fat vegetable or chicken broth. Simmer until the vegetables are soft, then purée the mixture in a blender. Return to the saucepan and add herbs and spices to taste. To make soups healthier yet, add cooked lentils, beans, or other legumes.

LOW-FAT DRINKS
Try a shake made from low-fat yogurt, banana, orange juice, and honey. Or simply blend fruits of your choice with orange or apple juice for a dairy-free shake.

OSTEOPOROSIS

Osteoporosis, or loss of bone mass, occurs in both men and women throughout adult life. With increasing age, more calcium is lost than replaced, leading to diminished bone density.

Protein and bone loss

Several studies have suggested that a diet high in protein causes the body to excrete calcium in the urine. Therefore a regular intake of excess protein will accelerate bone loss. It is recommended that you make high-protein foods only a small part of each meal and fill up with starchy foods, fruits, and vegetables instead.

Women are more prone to osteoporosis than men because they have less bone mass to begin with and rapid bone loss occurs after menopause, when levels of the hormone estrogen fall sharply. A British study of 182 pairs of postmenopausal twins, published in 1995, suggests genetic predisposition may also play a role in osteoporosis.

HOW BONE LOSS OCCURS

The skeleton is continually in a dynamic state throughout adult life. As bone wears away and new bone forms, its calcium is recycled. With age and hormonal changes, bones become brittle and weak. Many sufferers complain of bone pain, particularly in the hips and back. Some become stooped, a condition known as dowager's hump, from a weakening of the spine.

WOMEN AND OSTEOPOROSIS

Estrogen helps maintain bone density in women. If this hormone declines because of diseased ovaries or severe underweight, bone density will be lost.

After menopause, when estrogen naturally declines, bone mass is rapidly lost. Maintaining an adequate calcium intake throughout adult life will slow this loss. However, women at greater risk through a family history of osteoporosis are advised to take hormone replacement therapy.

OTHER RISK FACTORS

Race is an important factor. Africans have denser bones than north Europeans and are at less risk, while Asians and Hispanics have lower-density bones and are at greater risk. Adequate physical activity and calcium intake can overcome this predisposition.

THE FINE BALANCE BETWEEN BONE GROWTH AND LOSS

The calcium in your bones is constantly being dissolved and replaced as mineral levels in the blood drop and the body demands that they be replenished.

With age and changes in hormone levels, such as occur during menopause, calcium depletion begins to outweigh regeneration and the bones become weakened.

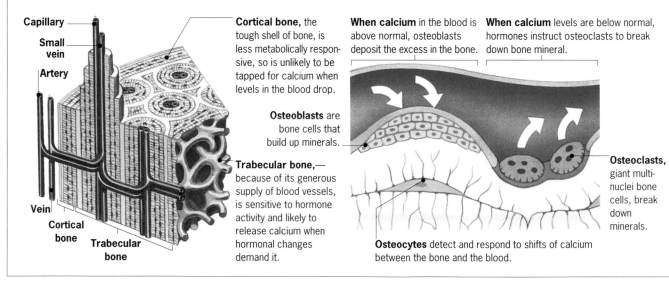

Capillary

Small vein

Artery

Vein

Cortical bone

Trabecular bone

Cortical bone, the tough shell of bone, is less metabolically responsive, so is unlikely to be tapped for calcium when levels in the blood drop.

Osteoblasts are bone cells that build up minerals.

Trabecular bone,— because of its generous supply of blood vessels, is sensitive to hormone activity and likely to release calcium when hormonal changes demand it.

When calcium in the blood is above normal, osteoblasts deposit the excess in the bone.

When calcium levels are below normal, hormones instruct osteoclasts to break down bone mineral.

Osteoclasts, giant multi-nuclei bone cells, break down minerals.

Osteocytes detect and respond to shifts of calcium between the bone and the blood.

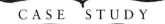

A Changing Woman

As women approach menopause, they often become conscious of age-related diseases. The risk of developing osteoporosis, for instance, is greatly increased because of the dramatic reduction in estrogen, which aids in calcium absorption. Dietary measures taken early in life will reduce this risk, particularly if there is a family history of osteoporosis.

Lisa, a 30-year-old marketing director, is married to John. Recently her grandmother was diagnosed with osteoporosis, and Lisa has since learned that a family history of the disease increases her chances of being affected. She knows that a calcium-rich diet is vital for staving off osteoporosis. Before hearing about her grandmother, Lisa had cut down on high-calorie foods, particularly dairy products, to avoid putting on weight. Now she is worried that she may have put herself at risk. On visiting her doctor to discuss her fears, she was assured that at her age she is still able to influence the chances of maintaining strong post-menopausal bones; he advised her on dietary and exercise measures.

WHAT SHOULD LISA DO?

First Lisa must maintain an adequate intake of calcium-rich foods. Low-fat and nonfat dairy products will help her avoid excess calories. She should also eat green vegetables, beans, and fish with bones, such as sardines. The fish supply not only calcium but also vitamin D, needed for calcium absorption. Calcium is not the only factor; magnesium, which Lisa can obtain from green vegetables, whole grains, nuts, poultry, meat, and eggs, is important in protecting bones. Lisa should minimize her caffeine intake, which can interfere with calcium absorption, and moderate her sugar and salt. It is also essential that she exercise regularly, taking a 20-minute brisk walk daily, for example.

Action Plan

FAMILY
Visit doctor to determine real risk of osteoporosis. Ask about a bone density test and whether such a test would be useful.

DIET
Increase intake of green vegetables and low-fat dairy products. Drink less coffee, particularly with meals. Cut down on sugary snacks.

EXERCISE
Walk to and from the station instead of taking the bus, and walk up stairs rather than using an escalator or elevator. Participate in sports on the weekends.

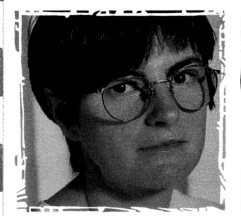

FAMILY
Women who have a family history of osteoporosis should take extra care to protect themselves.

DIET
Eating high-calcium foods before, during, and after menopause is one way to protect against bone loss.

EXERCISE
Lack of regular weight-bearing exercise can add to bone loss, increasing the risk of osteoporosis.

HOW THINGS TURNED OUT FOR LISA

Lisa changed her diet after consulting a nutritionist and found ways to increase calcium intake without extra fat. John joined her in her new diet and set up a weekly tennis game. After six months Lisa felt fitter, healthier, and confident that her new lifestyle would help stave off osteoporosis. The doctor assures her that future bone loss will be a natural result of aging and not pose a serious health risk if she maintains her new habits.

Supplements that don't help

Avoid taking bonemeal as a calcium supplement because it is not well absorbed and may contain toxic substances. Similarly, oyster shell, sold as a calcium supplement, is not well absorbed by the digestive system. A calcium-magnesium supplement called dolomite may also contain toxic substances, such as lead and mercury; it, too, is not easily absorbed and, in fact, may interfere with the absorption of other minerals in the body.

Weight-bearing exercise, such as aerobics or brisk walking, is essential for maintaining bone mass because it encourages bone building. Smoking and heavy drinking of alcohol may contribute to the early onset of osteoporosis because they increase calcium losses from the body.

PREVENTION MUST START EARLY

During the period of rapid growth in adolescence, bone deposition is at its greatest. An adequate calcium supply at this stage ensures maximum bone density. Recommended daily intakes of calcium are 1,200 to 1,500 mg per day for adolescents and young adults. Rich sources of calcium include milk, cheese, yogurt, canned sardines, and most leafy greens. Some breads, orange juice, and other foods fortified with calcium are also good sources. It is particularly important for women to maintain an adequate intake of calcium throughout adult life. Recommended daily intake for adult women is 800 to 1,200 mg before menopause, 1,000 to 1,500 afterward.

An adequate supply of vitamin D is also needed for calcium absorption. The action of sunlight on the skin is an excellent source of vitamin D. Food sources include oily fish, eggs, and fortified margarine.

Young people should be encouraged to exercise regularly because this increases bone density. Bones grow stronger if subjected to the various stresses and strains imposed during physical activity.

FACTORS THAT AFFECT CALCIUM STATUS

With excessive caffeine consumption, calcium is excreted in the urine. It is best to limit coffee and other caffeinated drinks to two cups or glasses a day. Excessive amounts of protein and sodium also accelerate excretion of calcium. To best absorb calcium, your body also needs vitamin D, found in some fortified milk products, margarine, and butter; oily fish; and egg yolks.

It is known that some high-fiber foods, including wheat bran, brown rice, and other whole grains, contain phytates, which tend to bind with calcium and prevent its absorption. However, many experts believe that it takes very large quantities for this to be a problem. Spinach, Swiss chard, almonds, rhubarb, and chocolate all contain oxalic acid, another compound that binds with calcium to form a salt that the body can't use, but it fortunately affects the absorption of calcium only from that particular food.

Steroids used to treat severe asthma, chronic bronchitis, and rheumatoid arthritis can also accelerate bone loss. Supplements of calcium and vitamin D given in such cases can help to maintain calcium status.

WHAT ABOUT SUPPLEMENTS?

Some people, including vegans, pregnant women, and those who have severe allergies, cannot easily maintain sufficient calcium intake through diet alone. For them, supplements may be necessary. However, it is important to discuss supplementation with a doctor first. Some people develop constipation from calcium supplements. Also, taking excessive amounts may cause kidney stones in susceptible people. Calcium supplements can be toxic in large doses, especially those that contain vitamin D, and may also interfere with iron absorption.

Calcium supplements come in many forms. The most popular and inexpensive is calcium carbonate, which also contains the largest percentage of calcium. Calcium citrate is the most easily absorbed but more expensive;. Calcium phosphate, calcium gluconate, and calcium lactate are also available.

Calcium carbonate and calcium phosphate supplements are best absorbed if taken 1 to 1½ hours after a meal with a full glass of water. In general, calcium is better absorbed from food sources than from supplements, and there are fewer risks of toxicity.

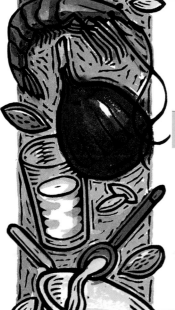

CALCIUM IN AND OUT

Diet can boost calcium intake, but other factors may deplete it. The cumulative effects are important, so increase foods on the left and decrease factors on the right.

CALCIUM-RICH FOODS	CALCIUM DEPLETERS
Milk and dairy products	Caffeine
Tofu	Alcohol
Soft bones of canned fish	Phytate-rich foods
Dried legumes	Oxalate-rich foods
Most dark leafy greens	Smoking
Some fortified foods	Lack of exercise

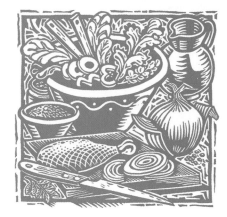

CHAPTER 3

HEALING COMPONENTS OF FOOD

A large body of mounting evidence suggests that there are many compounds in foods that have the potential to protect against some diseases, notably cancer. Previously scientists concentrated on the nutrients in foods already known to be essential—the vitamins and minerals. But now there is growing interest in other compounds that may not be essential for the body to function properly but might boost defences against illness.

THE HEALING POWER OF PLANTS

The majority of edible plants are packed with healthy elements. Some, known as phytochemicals, are specific to plants, while others—vitamins and minerals—are shared with animal sources.

Phytochemicals, literally "plant chemicals," are present in all fruits and vegetables. They include antioxidants, which are known to destroy carcinogens. Phytochemicals have healing qualities, both for preventing and for treating disease.

Although they do not perform specific functions in the body the way that vitamins and minerals do, phytochemicals appear to play a role in preventing degenerative conditions such as cancer and heart disease. Evidence is inconclusive about how they work, but it seems clear that people who consume a diet rich in fruits and vegetables have lower rates of degenerative diseases.

FREE RADICALS

It has been suggested that certain phytochemicals help protect the body from harmful substances called free radicals. These are by-products of normal metabolic processes in the body, such as digesting food, but they are also produced by cigarette smoke, environmental pollutants like car exhaust fumes, X-rays, and radiation from the sun.

Like a power station, your body burns fuel from food in order to release energy. During this process free radicals are generated. These are also produced by immune cells in response to invading bacteria and viruses. Left unchecked, free radicals can disturb the intricate mechanism of body cells and damage their DNA and other genetic material.

As part of its defense mechanism, the body produces protective enzymes that effectively neutralize free radicals before they can damage cells. But over time the effects of oxidation can accumulate, thus increasing the possibility of the body developing degenerative disorders and tumors.

ANTIOXIDANTS

Plants also contain defense mechanisms against oxidation. These are the antioxidants in fresh fruits and vegetables, which are believed to boost protection against free radicals in humans. Hundreds of studies are underway to examine their functions.

Antioxidant vitamins

Beta carotene, the plant form of vitamin A, is present in all brightly colored fruits and vegetables such as cantaloupes, red and yellow peppers, mangoes, carrots, and leafy green vegetables. These foods also provide
continued on page 53

THE FREE-RADICAL REACTION

Each antioxidant, no matter what its source, has a specific role to play in countering the effects of free radicals. In order to achieve the fullest protection, you should eat foods regularly that include both vitamin and mineral antioxidants.

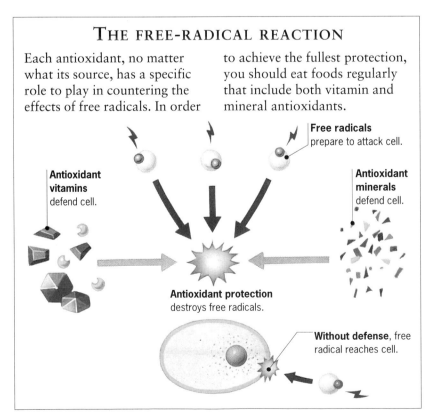

Free radicals prepare to attack cell.

Antioxidant vitamins defend cell.

Antioxidant minerals defend cell.

Antioxidant protection destroys free radicals.

Without defense, free radical reaches cell.

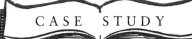
A Man Who Is Often Ill

Everybody knows someone who is always ill or who seems unable to throw off an infection as easily as everyone else. Coughs, colds, flu, cystitis, abscesses, bronchitis—all these problems can occur more frequently when the immune system is run down, which in turn may be the result of an inadequate diet.

Brian is a 68-year-old retiree who lives alone. He can no longer afford to eat the way he used to, and for weeks at a time he is depressed and lives largely on toast and coffee or tea. In the past five years, Brian has had bronchitis every winter and frequent attacks of pleurisy—a very painful inflammation of the lungs. Although Brian's doctors are very concerned about him, they have never considered referring him for nutritional counseling because these illnesses are not considered to be diet-related. Brian's friends worry about him, but Brian attributes his illness to his age and awaits warmer months to clear his chest problems. A friend who was helped by nutritional advice urges Brian to see a nutritionist.

WHAT SHOULD BRIAN DO?

Brian's nutritionist advises him to change his diet to incorporate foods that are rich sources of the antioxidants (see page 50) and other nutrients that Brian's immune system desperately needs.

Brian has never tried to cook for himself; he generally eats expensive take-out and packaged foods, so the first thing he must do is buy some cooking equipment. One of his friends offers to lend him the money and help him buy what he needs.

Next, Brian must visit his local supermarket to buy vegetables and fruits, whole-grain bread, brown rice, lentils, and dried beans; then he must follow instructions the nutritionist has given him for preparing simple meals.

Action Plan

EATING HABITS
For the first month or two, plan shopping and weekly menus in advance in order to establish a new cooking and eating routine.

PERSONAL HEALTH
Keep to a simple, healthy eating routine, which will help prevent added stress caused by illness.

FINANCES
Check local supermarkets each week for the best buys in fresh foods. Go often so there isn't too much to carry and the produce is fresh. Don't buy foods that are obviously in poor condition.

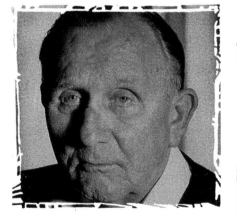

FINANCES
Some people worry that eating healthfully will prove to be very expensive.

EATING HABITS
Illnesses that do not initially appear to be diet related may in fact stem from a weakening of the immune system due to poor nutrition.

PERSONAL HEALTH
Long-term stress can lead to depression and a failure to look after yourself properly. In turn, poor nutrition and illness can worsen depression.

HOW THINGS TURNED OUT FOR BRIAN

Brian's friends helped with his new routine. He was surprised to find that the recommended foods were cheaper than the prepared foods he was using before. The low cost of the diet helped reduce stress; soon he noticed renewed energy. That winter Brian had a mild case of bronchitis but no pleurisy. As his cooking confidence grew, he invited friends for dinner. Brian feels that his new diet has helped make him a new man.

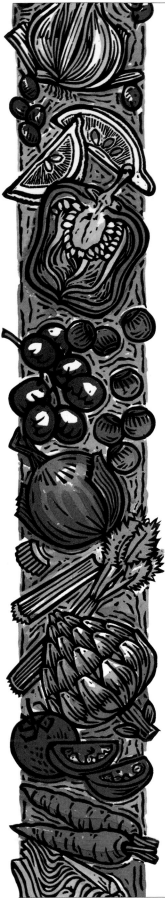

PHYTOCHEMICALS

Of the thousands of phytochemicals that exist, dozens are currently being investigated. Some of the better-known ones are listed below, with their main food sources and the possible roles they play in health maintenance and the fight against disease.

PHYTOCHEMICAL	GOOD SOURCES	ROLE IN HEALTH
Carotenoids	All brightly colored fruits and vegetables	Beta carotene is converted into vitamin A by the body. Like other carotenoids, such as lutein and lycopene, it is a potent antioxidant that mops up free radicals and may protect the body against cancer.
Flavonoids	Many fruits and vegetables, including onions, kale, celery, apples, and cranberries; also tea, coffee, and red wine	Flavonoids have an antioxidant action in the body. There is an association between a high intake of flavonoids and a decreased risk of cancer and heart disease. High consumption of green tea in the Far East and red wine in France may be responsible for lower rates of certain chronic diseases in those countries.
Isothiocyanates	Kohlrabi, broccoli, and cabbage	These compounds may prevent carcinogens, or cancer-causing substances, from forming in the body and may also help break them down once they are formed.
Indoles	Broccoli, cabbage, Brussels sprouts, and kale	May protect against cancer by preventing carcinogens from damaging the genetic material of body cells. Indoles are also thought to protect against certain forms of hormone-dependent breast cancer. They stimulate the breakdown of the female hormone estrogen in the liver, so that less of it is then available to help a tumor grow.
Ellagic acid	Grapes and nuts	May detoxify potentially carcinogenic substances in the body.
Cynarin	Artichokes	Some evidence suggests that cynarin may help reduce blood cholesterol levels and generally improve liver function. Although this has not been substantiated scientifically, many health food stores sell preparations containing cynarin.
Phytoestrogens	Soybeans, tofu, and other soy products	These substances are similar to the female hormone estrogen, but they are much weaker. Phytoestrogens may protect against atherosclerosis by exerting an estrogenic effect and may also protect against certain forms of hormone-dependent breast cancer. They compete with female estrogen, which is needed for tumors to grow, thus minimizing its negative effects.
Sulfur-containing compounds	Garlic and onions	Garlic has long been reputed to have antibacterial and antiviral properties. Certain compounds present in garlic may also reduce levels of blood cholesterol and decrease the risk of cancer by inhibiting the formation of carcinogens. Onions, from the same family, are widely believed to have a similar effect.
Coumarins	Tomatoes, green peppers, and carrots	These may inhibit the formation of carcinogens in the gut, thereby protecting against stomach cancer.

vitamin C, another antioxidant. One large mango or half a red pepper supplies the daily requirement of vitamin C for an adult. Citrus fruits, strawberries, and kiwi fruits are also rich in this vitamin.

Vitamin E is another antioxidant that prevents free radicals from attacking body cells. It is found in wheat germ, vegetable oils such as sunflower and corn oil, as well as avocados, nuts, and seeds.

Although evidence for the protective effect of antioxidants is growing, there is no accepted recommendation on daily intake. Current advice, however, is that you should eat five to seven servings of vegetables and fruits a day rather than take supplements.

Flavonoids

In addition to essential vitamins, fruits and vegetables contain an array of other potentially beneficial substances that may exert antioxidant action in the body. Some, such as flavonoids, also known as bioflavonoids, are being investigated currently by nutrition scientists. Although this is an area of great debate, the evidence so far looks promising. Flavonoids are found in such foods as cranberries, onions, kale, broccoli, apples, red wine, and tea. The flavonoids in red wine are thought to protect against atherosclerosis.

Antioxidant minerals

Some minerals found in both plant and animal foods also have properties that assist the body's defenses. These are essential components of some antioxidant enzymes produced in the body. Enzymes are substances that promote specific biochemical processes. They act as catalysts, helping to convert one substance into another one without being affected themselves.

Selenium is an integral component of the enzyme glutathione peroxidase, which neutralizes free radicals in the body. In times of illness, stress, or exposure to toxins such as cigarette smoke, the body uses more selenium; thus a good intake is needed to ensure adequate production of glutathione peroxidase. Brazil nuts are an excellent source of selenium, but it is also found in seafood, lean meats, whole grains, eggs, and beans.

Other minerals

Copper is a component of many enzymes, including superoxide dismutase, which neutralizes free radicals in the body. Nuts and seeds are good sources of copper. Zinc, manganese, and iron are also important. Green vegetables and whole-grain cereals are moderate sources of zinc and iron, and nuts, cereals, and legumes are rich in manganese.

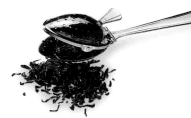

FLAVONOIDS IN TEA
A particularly rich source of flavonoids is green tea. Japan, where green tea consumption is high, has a relatively low rate of heart disease. Black tea also contains flavonoids, and a Dutch study in 1995 reported lower rates of heart disease among Dutch men with a high intake of flavonoids from onions, apples, and black tea. In Great Britain, tea consumption is also high, but so is heart disease. It could be that the benefits of tea there are neutralized by the addition of milk, which may bind with flavonoids to prevent their absorption.

SOURCES OF ANTIOXIDANT MINERALS

Antioxidant minerals can be found in a variety of food sources, particularly shellfish and nuts. Other mineral-rich foods include liver, poultry, whole-grain breads, fortified cereals, legumes, and dried fruits. A well-balanced eating plan should offer all the minerals that your body needs.

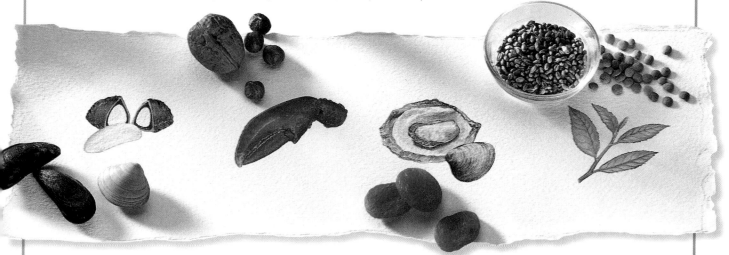

Selenium is plentiful in Brazil nuts and shellfish. Other good sources include legumes and whole grains.

Copper is plentiful in crustaceans, such as lobster, and many nuts; liver and legumes are also good sources.

Zinc and iron-rich foods include shellfish, such as oysters and clams, and dried apricots.

Manganese can be found in tea and coffee, also in various grains and legumes.

HEALING ANIMAL FOODS

Although most health experts recommend that consumption of animal products be limited, many beneficial components found in animal foods help prevent disease.

Eating yogurt

Many yogurts are high in saturated fat, so save them for special treats and buy low-fat and nonfat varieties for everyday use. For extra nutrients you can add your own fresh or dried fruit and nuts or seeds to plain yogurt. The yogurts with live bacteria are more effective at helping your body fight certain kinds of infections.

FISH OILS
The omega-3 fatty acids found in oily fish, such as herring and salmon, have been shown to provide vital help in the battle against heart disease.

Both plant and animal foods contain many of the same nutrients, but there are two that are found mainly in animal foods—vitamin B_{12} and omega-3 fatty acids. The first exists in all animal products, including meat, fish, milk, and eggs. The second is found primarily in fish, especially cold-water varieties. Vegans, who eat no animal foods, may be deficient in these two elements and should find fortified sources or take supplements in consultation with a doctor.

OILY FISH

Omega-3 fatty acids, which are found in abundance in oily fish such as salmon, mackerel, and bluefish, can reduce the risk of coronary heart disease by decreasing the viscosity, or stickiness, of the blood. People who eat a lot of fish, such as the Inuit Eskimos, have blood that does not clot as easily as the blood of groups of people who consume small amounts of fish. This is particularly helpful in preventing thrombosis.

A two-year British study on 2,033 men published in 1989 clearly showed a reduced mortality in men who had already had a heart attack and started consuming oily fish or taking fish oil supplements twice a week. Although the current recommendation for oily fish consumption is two servings a week, some experts suggest it should be even more.

Fish oils can be helpful for rheumatoid arthritis. Two or three servings of oily fish a week reduces the inflammatory response in the joints of some sufferers. Oily fish include fresh tuna (not canned, as the beneficial oils are removed) and fresh or canned salmon, sardines, trout, and mackerel.

YOGURT AND BACTERIA

Yogurt is considered a wonder food in many parts of the world, and recent research suggests it is indeed beneficial for health. It is made by adding a starter culture (bacteria) to pasteurized milk, then storing it in a warm place until it sets. The culture contains friendly lactic acid bacteria, such as *Lactobacillus bulgaricus* and *Lactobacillus acidophilus*. These ferment the milk sugar lactose to lactic acid, which gives yogurt its sour taste.

These friendly bacteria are believed to help fight yeast infections such as candidiasis, as well as harmful bacteria in the gut. Yogurt is often recommended as a topical treatment for candidiasis. The friendly bacteria in yogurt are also claimed to be able to aid digestion by restoring the useful bacteria in the stomach, which may be depleted or destroyed by antibiotics.

ZINC, IRON, AND COPPER

Although zinc, iron, and copper—essential to the building of red blood cells, the proper functioning of numerous enzymes, and many other bodily processes—are found in some plants, they are most abundant in animal foods and are most easily absorbed from them. Liver, red meat, and seafood are the best sources.

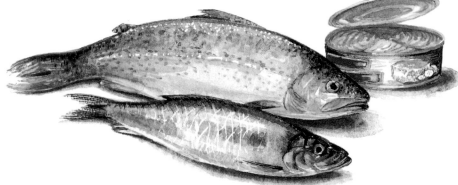

THREE SPECIAL DIETS AND THEIR BENEFITS

There is plenty of evidence that the diets in Mediterranean countries and Japan are beneficial in ways that the typical North American diet is not. A vegetarian diet also has health benefits.

It can be helpful when considering a change in diet to look for inspiration at the eating habits and general health of other cultures. Adopting the best aspects of such diets can provide variety in your meals and actively benefit your health.

THE MEDITERRANEAN DIET

The Mediterranean diet has received a lot of attention in recent years because the occupants of countries such as Greece, Spain, Italy, and Turkey have much lower rates of coronary artery disease than people in North America and northern Europe.

A typical midday or evening meal in a Mediterranean country consists of pasta, rice, or grains such as couscous (semolina wheat in the form of granules) served with vegetables or seafood and accompanied by salad and bread. The meal is most often concluded with fresh fruit.

Because of the prominence of fruits and vegetables, the Mediterranean diet provides more fiber than some other diets. Dietary fiber helps maintain regular bowel function and is thought to protect against some forms of cardiovascular disease and cancer. Health experts recommend consuming between 20 and 35 grams of fiber daily from a variety of foods, including whole-grain breads and cereals, dried legumes, nuts, seeds, and all kinds of fruits and vegetables.

Although the Mediterranean diet is relatively high in total fat, sometimes more than the 30 percent maximum recommended by nutritionists in this country, it comes mainly from olives and olive oil, which are high in monounsaturated fat. Unlike saturated fat, the fat in olive oil does not raise blood cholesterol. In fact, it has been shown to lower LDLs ("bad" cholesterol) and raise HDLs.

THE JAPANESE DIET

Japan has one of the lowest rates of heart disease among affluent countries, and diet is thought to be a key. Although total fat is about 30 percent, the Japanese diet is generally high in polyunsaturated fats from soy products and relatively high in omega-3 fatty acids from oily fish.

Fruit and vegetable intake, however, is similar to that in North America. Yet something in the Japanese diet apparently compensates in some measure for the lower levels of dietary fiber.

Low rates of breast cancer in the East have been attributed to the soy-rich diet. Soybeans contain high levels of phytoestrogens, which may interfere with the ability of the body's estrogen to promote the growth of certain kinds of tumors (see page 52).

The Japanese, however, suffer from high rates of stomach cancer, possibly because of a high salt intake and the prevalence in their diet of large quantities of smoked, pickled, and cured foods. Salted fish is a traditional part of the diet in Japan and besides being a risk factor for cancer, salt raises blood pressure and the risk of stroke. If you follow a Japanese diet, cut back on the high-salt ingredients or preparations.

The effect of green tea on Japanese health has also been the focus of scientific interest (see page 53).

THE VEGETARIAN DIET

As a group, vegetarians clearly enjoy certain health advantages. For one thing, they tend to have lower cholesterol levels (vegans, who eat no animal foods, have the lowest) and are less likely to develop hypertension than meat eaters. Also, obesity, constipation, and diverticulosis are rare among people who

THE MEDITERRANEAN DIET A plentitude of fruits and vegetables and a generous use of olive oil are two factors that make this diet healthful.

THE JAPANESE DIET Fish and soy products, both low in saturated fat, are good staples for a healthy diet. Green tea also has benefits.

consume a high-fiber plant-based diet that is also low in fat. Some vegetarian diets, however, can be high in saturated fat from whole-milk dairy foods. Also, anemia can be a problem for vegetarians because the iron in plant foods is more difficult to absorb, and a high intake of dairy products can further decrease the body's ability to absorb iron. Eating more fruits and vegetables rich in vitamin C increases the amount of iron absorbed from plant foods.

Meat eaters who want to obtain the benefits of a vegetarian diet should substitute at least some of their weekly meat intake with vegetables and protein-rich beans, grains, and nuts. If this is too difficult, at least part of the meat intake should be replaced with fish, particularly oily fish such as salmon.

THE VEGETARIAN DIET
A well-balanced vegetarian diet that includes low-fat dairy products and a wide variety of fruits, vegetables, and complex carbohydrates can help combat heart disease and many cancers.

Pathway to health

The French traditionally consume a diet high in saturated fat from meat, butter, cream, and cheese, yet they have a heart-attack rate one-third that of Americans. This surprising fact has become known as the French paradox and has been linked to the high consumption of red wine in France. Researchers have not determined what the preventive factor is. Theories advanced are that flavonoids in wine (see page 82) are responsible; wine with meals may reduce clot formation; moderate wine consumption may raise levels of HDLs ("good" cholesterol).

HEALTH AND YOUR DIET

Certain aspects of a diet may help prevent some diseases and disorders, while others in that same diet may promote health problems. The best approach is to incorporate the positive aspects of each diet and reap all their benefits.

DISEASE	MEDITERRANEAN DIET	JAPANESE DIET	VEGETARIAN DIET
Heart disease	✔ High intake of complex carbohydrates, fruits, and vegetables	✔ High intake of fish oils and antioxidants from green tea	✔ High intake of complex carbohydrates, fruits, and vegetables
High blood cholesterol	✔ Monounsaturated fat in olive oil	✔ Low in total fat, particularly saturated fat	✘ Possible high intake of saturated fat from dairy products
Stroke		✘ High intake of salt in smoked, pickled, and salted food	
Cancers general	✔ Antioxidant nutrients from fruits, vegetables, and red wine	✔ Antioxidants from green tea	✔ Antioxidant nutrients from fruits and vegetables and low saturated fat from meat-free diet
breast		✔ Phytoestrogens in soy-rich diet	
stomach		✘ High intake of salt	
bowel	✔ High dietary fiber from fruits and vegetables	✘ Low dietary fiber, fewer fruits and vegetables	✔ High dietary fiber from fruits and vegetables
Anemia	✔ Good iron intake from meat and seafood		✘ Decreased absorption of iron from excess milk

✔ A check denotes an aspect of the diet that may help protect against the disorder.

✘ A cross denotes an aspect of the diet that may exacerbate the disorder.

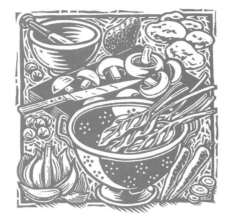

CHAPTER 4

SUPERFOODS

Certain foods, or groups of food, can be deemed superfoods because they contain high levels of essential nutrients. They do not exert their beneficial effects in isolation—no one food contains all the nutrients that your body needs—but if included regularly and in sufficient amounts in a well-balanced diet, they can lead to optimum health.

VEGETABLES AND FRUITS

Low in fat and high in vitamins, minerals, and fiber, vegetables and fruits are also wonderfully versatile. Both raw and cooked, they can easily become a major part of a healthy eating plan.

Eye protection

Research suggests that beta carotene and other related constituents in orange and yellow fruits and vegetables and green leafy vegetables may reduce the risk of developing vision disorders. Surveys carried out in the United States and Finland showed that diets rich in vitamins C and E and beta carotene reduced the risk of cataract formation. The best protection appeared to occur when dark green vegetables were eaten four to five times a week.

Around the world vegetables and fruits are recognized for their versatility—there are hundreds of varieties, and new ones are being developed every day. They are also appreciated for their healthfulness, supplying most of the vitamins, minerals, and fiber that the body needs.

ROOT VEGETABLES

Root vegetables, including carrots, turnips, beets, and rutabagas, are storehouses of energy and nutrients. Among them, carrots earn the title of superfood because they contain an abundance of beta-carotene, the orange-yellow pigment found in numerous vegetables and fruits that is just one of many compounds known as the carotenoids. Beta carotene is converted in the body to vitamin A, essential for healthy eye function and normal growth and development. (One carrot provides more than six times the recommended daily

allowance of vitamin A.) A powerful antioxidant, beta carotene also plays an important role in the fight against cancer.

Carrots and health

Low intakes of beta-carotene have been linked with an increased incidence of some cancers. A large study conducted in Italy in 1986 demonstrated (after accounting for other factors such as smoking) that people who did not eat carrots were twice as likely to develop lung cancer as those who consumed them once a week or more.

Carrots are also a useful source of dietary fiber, particularly soluble fiber, which has been shown to lower blood cholesterol levels. Thus they may offer protection against the development of heart disease and possibly cancer, particularly of the colon.

Buying and storing guide

Choose firm, brightly colored roots. Avoid carrots that are cracked or very dry or have bruised areas or dark spots on the roots or mold around the tops. Store them in the refrigerator in a perforated plastic bag; remove the tops before storing.

GREEN LEAFY VEGETABLES

They come in many varieties, but green leafy vegetables can be grouped because of the common range of essential nutrients

HOW BETA CAROTENE HELPS TO BEAT CANCER

A powerful antioxidant within body cells, beta carotene has been found to be particularly effective in reducing the risk of lung cancer and has been linked also to protection against cancers of the bladder, cervix, and lining of the uterus. It is also believed to prevent the formation of nitrosamines (possible carcinogens) in the stomach.

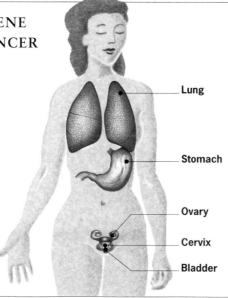

- Lung
- Stomach
- Ovary
- Cervix
- Bladder

they contain. Most leafy greens—spinach, beet greens, and dandelion greens especially, but also arugula, chicory, and Swiss chard—provide vitamins A, C, and E plus calcium in useful amounts. These three vitamins are powerful antioxidants that protect cells from attacks by free radicals.

In addition, leafy greens are usually excellent sources of iron and folic acid (folate), both of which are essential for healthy red blood cells. Evidence is emerging that folic acid may also be a protective factor against heart disease. It breaks down an amino acid called homocysteine, which can clog arteries.

Buying and storing guide
When buying greens, choose fresh leaves with a dark, rich color. Dry them as much as possible, pack them loosely in a plastic bag, and store them in the vegetable bin of the refrigerator. Use them within a few days; the longer they are stored, the more their nutrients, especially vitamin C, diminish.

CRUCIFEROUS VEGETABLES
The news has spread far and wide that cruciferous vegetables—among them broccoli, Brussels sprouts, cabbage, cauliflower, kale, and collards—are rich in bioflavonoids and other plant chemicals that protect against cancer. They are also good sources of the antioxidant vitamins C and A. Scientists believe that it is the combination of these antioxidants, plus dietary fiber and other constituents such as indoles (see page 52), that work together as anticancer agents. These plants also contain useful amounts of folate, iron, calcium, and other minerals.

Broccoli is the star of this group because it seems to have more cancer-fighting compounds than the others. People who eat broccoli regularly have fewer cancers of the colon, breast, cervix, lungs, prostate, esophagus, larynx, and bladder Recent studies also indicate that broccoli may improve lupus symptoms.

Buying and storing guide
Broccoli should have firm, strong stalks with bright green (or purple) flowers. Florets that are turning yellow are past their prime. Brussels sprouts should be firm and bright green; avoid any that have yellowing, wilted leaves or stalks. Cabbage should be firm and heavy, with crisp leaves.

FRUIT VEGETABLES
Some foods we consider vegetables are actually fruits, including peppers, tomatoes, and squashes. Sweet peppers, red ones in particular, qualify as superfoods. Ounce for ounce, they provide twice as much vitamin C as citrus fruits, and they are also high in beta carotene. Deeply colored peppers also contain bioflavonoids, thought to protect against cancer, and phenolic acids, which inhibit formation of cancer-causing nitrosamines.

The nutrient profile of the tomato speaks for itself: it contains all three antioxidant vitamins, A, C, and E, and therefore is an important anticancer vegetable. It also contains potassium, which helps regulate blood pressure, and another type of antioxidant called lycopene, which gives tomatoes their bright red color. Lycopene seems to enhance absorption of beta-carotene.

In some people an allergic reaction to tomatoes can cause mouth ulcers, eczema, headaches, indigestion, or heartburn. These people may find that cooked ones do not have the same effect as raw.

Squashes are divided generally into two types—summer and winter. The summer varieties are less nutrient dense because they are so high in water—about 95 percent. Most winter squashes are high in vitamin A, providing a whole day's allowance.

Buying and storing guide
Choose firm, unwrinkled peppers with a shiny, bright skin and clean, firm stalk. Store them, unwashed, in the bottom of the refrigerator; they will keep for 7 to 10 days.

Select firm tomatoes and avoid those with wrinkled skins. They always taste better if stored at room temperature but, once ripe, will keep only two to three days. They last up to two weeks stored in the refrigerator.

Summer squashes should be refrigerated. Most winter squashes will keep in a cool, dry place for up to three months.

THE VEGETABLE FACTOR Carrots, green leafy vegetables, peppers, cruciferous vegetables, and tomatoes are vital to a healthy diet.

NUTRIENT PROFILE OF A TOMATO

A 100-gram (3½-ounce) tomato contains one-third the adult RDA for vitamin C, three-fourths the RDA for vitamin A.

Vitamin C	20 mg
Vitamin A	820 IU
Vitamin E	1 mg
Energy	20 cal

BENEFICIAL BERRIES

Summer berries are particularly good, not to mention delicious, sources of vitamin C. They are also fine sources of soluble fiber, which helps to lower cholesterol levels and protects against heart disease. For centuries berries have been used as remedies for a number of conditions.

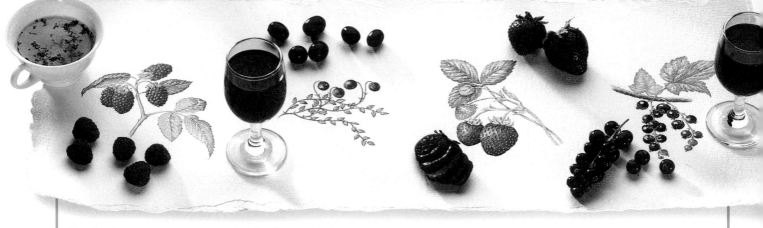

Raspberries are used to aid digestion, ease labor pains, and sometimes to reduce fevers.

Cranberries and blueberries may aid in recurring urinary tract infections by preventing bacteria from adhering to the bladder wall.

Strawberries are believed to aid digestion and, some say, are a powerful aphrodisiac.

Red currants help regulate blood pressure; black currants also relieve sore throats and diarrhea.

CITRUS FRUITS

Citrus fruits, including oranges, grapefruit, mandarin oranges, lemons, and tangerines, are well known for their vitamin C content. As a potent antioxidant, vitamin C mops up free radicals in the watery parts of cells. And it is also believed to enable vitamin E to perform its own antioxidant activity as well. In addition, vitamin C promotes wound healing, fights infections, and helps with the absorption of iron from cereal and plant food sources.

Citrus fruits also contain some calcium, thiamine (vitamin B_1), and pectin, a soluble fiber found in the membranes between segments. (Pectin is thought to help lower blood cholesterol.) They are excellent sources of potassium, too.

The juices of citrus fruits retain most of the vitamins and minerals (fresh-squeezed retains the most), but eating the flesh gives you the benefit of the fiber and folic acid.

Buying and storing guide

Choose fruits that feel heavy and are glossy; avoid those with coarsely grained or dry skins. Fruits should be firm but not too hard. Store citrus fruits in the refrigerator for up to two weeks or at room temperature for four to five days.

SOURCES OF VITAMIN C
Your daily vitamin C needs can be supplied by: one small orange or half of a green or red pepper.

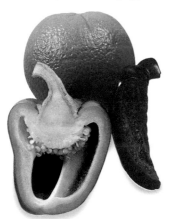

BERRIES

Berries are wonderfully versatile fruits, easy to eat out of hand, convenient storehouses of nutrients when dried, and a culinary pleasure in both sweet and savory dishes. For centuries many of them have also been used as remedies for various ailments (see above).

Berries vary in their essential nutrients, but most are good sources of vitamin C and potassium and also provide a fair amount of fiber. Strawberries contain more vitamin C than other berries or even citrus fruits. When fully ripe and in season, berries make wonderful low-calorie snacks. The calories climb rapidly when refined sugar is added for sweetening.

Buying and storing guide

If possible, buy berries when they are in season locally. Look for fruit that has a bright, uniform color, firm, unblemished skin, and clean, fresh stems. Eat berries immediately, or store them in the refrigerator, unwashed and uncovered, and eat as soon as possible.

APRICOTS

First cultivated in China about 4,000 years ago, fresh apricots are a low-calorie, delicious source of beta-carotene. When dried, however, their superfruit status (also calories) increases significantly. This is because drying concentrates the solid material of the fruit and the amount of fiber. High in soluble fiber and potassium, and a modest source of other minerals, including iron and calcium, dried apricots make a great snack.

Buying and storing guide
Buy fresh apricots in early summer, when they are plump and firm. Avoid damaged or over-soft fruit. Dried apricots and other dried fruits can be eaten without soaking. Fresh apricots can be stored in the refrigerator for up to a week; dried fruit should be stored in a cool, dry place.

BANANAS
Bananas are the perfect convenience food, a filling snack that is high in potassium, which is essential for healthy nerves and muscles and for regulating blood pressure. They are also high in natural sugars that give a healthy energy boost—many athletes eat them before competing.

Because bananas are easy to digest, they are an ideal early food for infants. They also soothe the digestive tract and for this reason are a good food to eat when recovering from a stomach upset or diarrhea; they are sometimes recommended as well for patients with ulcers. For these purposes they should always be completely ripe because unripe ones can actually cause stomach problems.

Buying and storing guide
Bananas are available all year round; ripe ones have a rich yellow, slightly mottled skin; any with dull, grayish skins will not ripen properly. Bananas continue to ripen when stored at room temperature. In the refrigerator they will turn black, but this does not affect their nutrient content or flavor.

PAPAYA
Papayas, too, are a good source of potassium, and they are rich in vitamins A and C; a medium-size papaya supplies more than three times the RDA for vitamin C. To prepare it for eating, cut it in half, remove the seeds, and squeeze a little fresh lime juice over the flesh to enhance its sweet flavor (and add a little more vitamin C).

Papaya contains an enzyme called papain, which is believed to have various healing properties. Papain is recommended as an aid to digestion (in Asia papaya seeds are

chewed to relieve stomachaches), and may help reduce the bloating and discomfort that some people experience after a large meal. In cooking, it is used as a tenderizer for meat.

Buying and storing guide
Available year-round, papayas are usually yellow or yellow-orange when fully ripe and give slightly when pressed. As a rule they are picked when only partly ripe; if you select one that is one-third to one-half yellow, it will ripen at room temperature in a few days. Use before it becomes soft or shriveled at the stem end.

KIWIFRUIT
Although relatively new in the Western diet, the kiwifruit merits special mention because it is higher in vitamin C than any other fruit—it contains about double the amount in a medium-size orange.

Buying and storing guide
A ripe kiwifruit is smooth and yields slightly to pressure; it is overripe when shriveled or mushy. Unripe kiwifruits can be stored for months as long as they are cold and away from other fruits. Keep them in a slightly open bag in the refrigerator. Store ripe ones the same way and they will last for several weeks.

AVOCADOS
Avocados contain vitamin E (an important antioxidant that protects the fatty parts of cells from free radical damage), a reasonable amount of fiber, beta carotene, folate, and more potassium than any other fruit.

Some people avoid avocados because they are relatively high in fat. However, half an avocado contains just over 100 calories, about the same as in a large banana, and of its 11 fat grams, over half are monounsaturated; they lower LDLs ("bad" cholesterol) and help protect against heart disease.

Buying and storing guide
Avocados are available all year round. Choose firm fruit and store it at room temperature until ripe, then keep it in the refrigerator and use within a few days. A sprinkling of lemon or lime juice will prevent cut avocado flesh from discoloring.

continued on page 64

PAPAIN
In medicin, the papaya enzyme papain is a component of spinal injections to ease the pain of slipped discs; it is used also in ointments to heal scarred or bruised skin.

Avocado news
Avocados harvested in winter have only one-third of the fat of those picked in autumn. This may be because the leaves of the avocado produce a hormone that prevents the fruit from ripening on the tree. There may be less of this hormone in the winter, when the leaves have dropped, so the fruit ripens more quickly.

Quicker winter ripening may also increase the percentage of sugar in the fruit and decrease the percentage of fat.

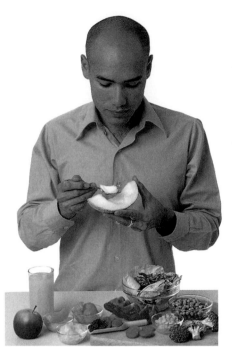

WHAT'S IN A SERVING
A single serving of fruit can be one medium-size apple, pear, or orange, ½ cup of diced fruit, or ¾ cup of fruit juice. One serving of vegetables is equal to 1 cup of raw leafy greens or ½ cup of cooked vegetables.

Breakfast: waffle, apricots, and yogurt

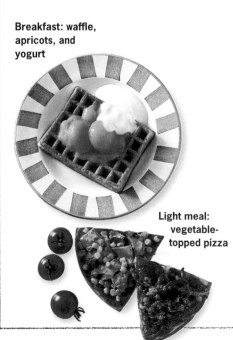

Light meal: vegetable-topped pizza

Ensuring an Adequate Intake of

Fruits and Vegetables

A diet that includes a variety of fruits and vegetables will boost your vitamin, mineral, and fiber intake and help protect you against fatigue and many illnesses and diseases.

FIVE-A-DAY FOR HEALTH

Many leading health organizations recommend consuming five to seven servings of fruits and vegetables every day. This includes juices, dried fruits, and frozen and canned fruits and vegetables, as well as fresh ones. Vegetarians may need even more servings to obtain enough nutrients. For many people this advice represents at least a 50 percent increase from current intake. A 1990 survey by the National Cancer Institute revealed that, on average, Americans eat fewer than two servings of vegetables a day, including salad, and often limit their choices to three or four varieties. Nature packages the vitamins, minerals, and fiber in plant foods in different proportions, so you need to eat a variety to maximize the benefits. Below are suggestions for incorporating vegetables and fruits readily into your daily meals.

FRUITS AND VEGETABLES THROUGHOUT THE DAY

Breakfast
- Add dried fruit, like prunes, dates, apricots, figs, or raisins, or fresh fruit, such as sliced strawberries, banana, or apple, to breakfast cereal.
- Add dried fruit to cooked cereal.
- Enjoy a bowl of cut-up mixed fruits, either on its own, or topped with plain or fruit yogurt.
- Make a fruit shake with any fresh fruit and yogurt or skim milk.
- Have a bowl of sliced banana in orange juice.
- Make a dried fruit compote with prunes, apricots, figs, raisins, and a little fruit juice or, in summer, a berry compote of seasonal berries.
- Serve pancakes or waffles with a warm fruit topping such as stewed apples, canned peaches or apricots (not those canned in syrup), or berries, and top with nonfat yogurt.

Lunch
- Enjoy puréed vegetable soups, such as carrot and ginger; spinach and potato; sweet red pepper; asparagus; watercress; or fennel and tomato.
- Cook extra vegetables for the evening meal, then toss them with a little salad dressing and add them to a sandwich the next day or use them to top a baked potato.
- Experiment with different salad combinations: avocado and orange; carrot and fennel; chickpea and tomato; peach, walnut, and cottage cheese; pepper and mushroom. Serve the above on a bed of leafy greens. Also consider grated carrot and zucchini tossed with lemon juice or sliced apples and pears with arugula.
- Top pizzas with a variety of sliced cooked vegetables; roasted vegetables are especially appealing.

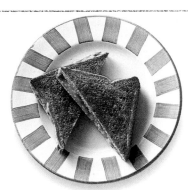

Snack time: peanut butter-banana sandwich

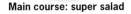

Main course: super salad

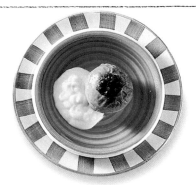

Dessert: baked apple with raisins and nuts

Snacks
• Fresh or dried fruit can be eaten any time of the day. Plan ahead so that you always have plenty of fresh fruit available.
• For a more substantial snack, try a banana and peanut butter sandwich, sliced apples and cinnamon toast, or a cheese and tomato sandwich.
• Fruit and vegetable purées make delicious dips. Try cooked and mashed root vegetable purées, such as carrot seasoned with coriander or curried parsnip and rutabaga and serve hot or cold with vegetable crudités.

Main courses
• Use hot puréed vegetables as sauces for meat, poultry, and fish. Try a puréed spinach, garlic, and herb sauce with chicken; chopped fresh tomato and basil sauce with fish; mushroom, shallot, and red wine sauce with beef or lamb.

• Add fruit to meat stews—for example, dried apricots with lamb; prunes with beef; cranberries with chicken; apple slices with pork.
• Add sliced raw vegetables or fruits to a dinner salad of mixed greens or spinach—for example, mushrooms, carrots, and peppers; kiwifruit and strawberries; pears and apples; oranges, onions, and black olives.
• Bake winter squash, such as Hubbard or acorn, with a stuffing of fresh bread crumbs and chopped dried apricots or cranberries.
• Replace the meat in lasagne and other pasta dishes with grated vegetables, such as zucchini, and legumes, such as peas, white kidney beans, or lentils.
• Bake red or green peppers with a stuffing of rice, kidney beans or chickpeas, and salsa, or chopped bread crumbs and tomatoes, seasoned with oregano and thyme.

Desserts
• With seasonal fruit, make crisps (sliced fruit baked with a topping of brown sugar, butter, fresh bread crumbs, and spices). Try peach and candied ginger, plum and pear, or apple and strawberry.
• For winter desserts, bake whole fruits, such as pears or apples, stuffing the centers with raisins and nuts and a sprinkling of spices.
• Top any combination of fresh, stewed, poached, or canned fruit with low-fat or nonfat frozen yogurt, sherbet, or sorbet.
• Fill kebab sticks with fresh, canned, or dried fruit and serve them cold, or grill them and top with a hot lemon sauce.
• Make your own fruit fools (puréed fruit and custard), using bananas and apricots, for example, or apples and raspberries, and topping with nonfat yogurt in place of the custard.

RETAINING VITAMINS AND MINERALS

• Buy fresh vegetables often and store them for as little time as possible. Nutrients diminish with each day of storage time.
• Prepare vegetables just before cooking them; do not soak them in water prior to cooking.
• Boil vegetables in a minimum of water and cook just long enough so they are tender but still slightly crisp.
• Use a minimum of salt in the cooking water; sodium destroys some of the nutrients.
• If you do have cooking water left, use it in a soup or add it to the cooking water for rice.

• Lightly steam, stir-fry, or microwave vegetables whenever possible to minimize vitamin losses.
• Serve cooked vegetables right away. Keeping them warm increases loss of vitamin C.
• Use frozen fruits and vegetables when their fresh versions are not in season. Except for a slight loss of vitamin C, they have as many nutrients as fresh ones and more than canned.

CLEANING FOODS
Whenever you can, wash or scrub vegetables rather than peeling them. Nutrients are more concentrated in or near the skin.

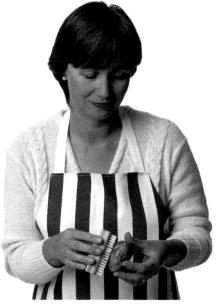

OTHER FRUITS

Apples, pears, and pineapples all have merits but vary in the useful amounts of vitamins A and C, fiber, potassium, and other nutrients that they contain.

Because of their soluble fiber, apples are recommended by naturopaths for relieving constipation, while stewed apples are often used during recovery from diarrhea, but the nutrients in apples are less than those of other fruits. The nutrients in pears are similar to those of apples but are more concentrated in the skin. Pears are also sweeter.

Pineapple is a good source of manganese, important for building strong bones, and it provides modest amounts of vitamin C. This tropical fruit also contains an enzyme called bromelain, which aids in digestion and has proved an effective anti-inflammatory for arthritis. Bromelain is also a meat tenderizer, and if applied to insect bites, it will help lessen the sting.

NUTRIENT PROFILE OF SUPER FRUITS AND VEGETABLES

The amounts of essential nutrients in different fruits and vegetables vary greatly. It is important to make choices that give you the widest possible benefits. Check the chart below for a selection that contains all the nutrients you need.

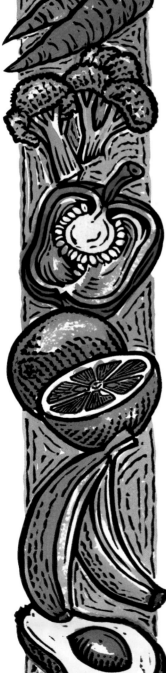

	BETA-CAROTENE	VITAMIN C	VITAMIN E	DIETARY FIBER	CALCIUM	IRON	FOLATE
FRUIT							
Apricots, fresh	✓✓			✓		✓	
dried	✓✓✓			✓	✓	✓✓	
Avocados	✓		✓	✓✓		✓	✓
Bananas		✓✓		✓			✓
Grapefruit		✓		✓			✓
Oranges		✓✓		✓	✓		✓
Papaya	✓✓✓	✓✓		✓			
Kiwifruits		✓✓✓		✓✓			✓
Raspberries		✓		✓✓			✓
Strawberries		✓✓		✓			✓
VEGETABLES							
Beet, roots				✓✓		✓	✓✓
tops	✓✓✓			✓		✓✓✓	✓
Broccoli	✓✓✓	✓✓✓		✓✓	✓✓	✓	✓✓
Brussels sprouts	✓✓	✓✓	✓	✓✓		✓	✓✓✓
Cabbage	✓	✓		✓		✓	✓
Carrots	✓✓✓			✓✓			
Peppers							
Green bell peppers	✓	✓✓✓		✓		✓	✓
Red bell peppers	✓✓✓	✓✓✓		✓		✓	✓
Spinach	✓✓✓	✓	✓✓	✓	✓	✓✓✓	✓✓✓
Squash							
Summer	✓			✓		✓	✓
Winter	✓✓			✓		✓	
Tomatoes	✓✓	✓	✓	✓		✓	✓

Compare the number of checks in the chart above against the figures shown below to find the levels of nutrients in an 80 g (3 oz) serving.

	✓✓✓	✓✓	✓
Beta-carotene	> 500 mcg	200–500 mcg	100–200 mcg
Vitamin C	> 100–150mg	50–100 mg	20–50 mg
Vitamin E	> 4 mg	2–4 mg	1–2 mg
Fiber	> 3–4 g	2–3 g	1–2 g
Calcium	> 150 mg	100–150 mg	50–100 mg
Iron	> 2 mg	1–2 mg	0.5–1 mg
Folate	> 100 mcg	50–100 mcg	15–50 mcg

STARCHY FOODS

Starches, found in a vast array of grains and vegetables, are major sources of energy. Nutritionists recommend that 55 to 65 percent of daily calories be supplied by starchy foods.

Staples in diets around the world, grains and starchy vegetables are energy providers. It is in the starch, or complex carbohydrate, where plants store their own energy, which is then broken down in the human body to form glucose.

An integral part of the complex carbohydrate in plants is fiber, itself a type of carbohydrate that makes up the cell walls. There are two types: soluble fiber, which is broken down in the large intestine and can help reduce blood cholesterol levels; and insoluble fiber, which is not broken down but passes through the large intestine unabsorbed. A lack of fiber in the diet can cause digestive disorders such as constipation (see page 105) and diverticulosis (see page 108). Whole-grain cereals provide both soluble and insoluble dietary fiber, thus helping to prevent constipation, protect against colon cancer, and reduce cholesterol levels.

STARCHES FROM GRAINS

Grains, or cereals—which include wheat, corn, oats, rice, kasha, millet, and barley—consist mainly of complex carbohydrates (starch) plus some protein and a small amount of fat. Except for vitamin B_{12}, unprocessed grains are a good source of all the B vitamins, which are concentrated in the outer layer of the seed; these vitamins can be severely depleted during milling along with the fiber. Grains also contain moderate amounts of calcium and iron.

Corn

Also known as maize, corn is a versatile plant. As a vegetable it is eaten fresh on the cob or its kernels can be frozen or canned for later consumption. Its dried, popped kernels are a popular snack, as are corn chips, and cornflakes have been a favorite breakfast cereal for years. Cornstarch serves as a thickener for gravies and puddings. Cornmeal is used to make polenta in Italy and tortillas in Mexico and is a staple in some African countries, where it is eaten as a porridge with meat or vegetable sauces. Cornmeal is ideal for celiac sufferers (see page 105) because it is gluten-free.

The nutritive value of the whole corn grain is similar to that of other cereals, with the main difference being corn's high content of beta carotene. Fresh corn on the cob should be eaten within one or two days of purchase. Frozen corn is an acceptable alternative and can be added to salads and stews.

Oats

Oat bran contains a significant amount of soluble fiber, which can help lower blood cholesterol levels. Soluble fiber is also useful for people with diabetes because it slows the rise of blood sugar levels after meals.

Oats are often associated with oatmeal or dry breakfast cereal, but they can be used in a number of other ways, for example, as a thickening agent in soups, to replace part of the wheat flour in cookie, cake, and muffin

Rolled oats
The popular oats for cooked breakfast cereal are available in two types: quick-cooking and old-fashioned. The second one is somewhat thicker, takes a little longer to cook, and has a slightly more pronounced texture. As a rule, the two are interchangable in recipes.

CEREALS
Oats, barley, rice, wheat, corn, and cornmeal are all excellent sources of starch and have the added bonus of being low in fat.

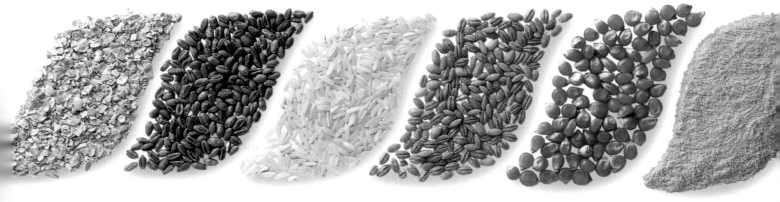

recipes, and as a filler in meat loaf. You do not have to eat oats to benefit from their goodness; a handful of oatmeal in your bath will soothe itchy or irritated skin.

Rice

More than half the world consumes rice as a dietary staple. Although this grain contains a little less protein than others, it is low in fat and is a good source of B vitamins. Much of the fiber, concentrated in the outer layer, is removed during milling, so white rice contains only one-third the fiber of brown. The B vitamins are also removed during milling, but most processors today enrich rice, thus restoring the vitamins.

Rice bran is even more effective than oat bran in lowering cholesterol levels. It is available in health food stores and is now being incorporated in many cereal products.

Breakfast cereals

Many grains are used in the production of ready-to-eat breakfast cereals, and an astonishing selection is available. Most of them are now fortified with vitamins (especially the B group) and minerals (especially iron) and provide an important source of these nutrients. Some cereals are also fortified with folic acid (folate), which is important for fetal development in early pregnancy.

The cereal box tells you how much of each nutrient is in the contents. Bran flakes have the highest fiber content and also the most iron. Unprocessed wheat bran is not the best way to increase fiber in the diet. Raw bran has a high content of phytic acid

that can bind with minerals such as calcium, iron, copper, and zinc and prevent them from being fully absorbed by the body.

Bread

Breads vary in nutritional content, depending on the kind, and the selections today are as numerous as those of breakfast cereals. Shoppers can find everything from simple white breads, in soft or crusty styles, to loaves containing seven grains and several types of seeds. Some breads—croissants and focaccia, for example—can be very high in fat and should be eaten only occasionally.

Although whole-grain breads are the best choice—most contain twice as much fiber as breads made with milled flours—white breads still remain the most popular. Fortunately, white bread has been made with enriched flour for many years now. This means that the iron and B vitamins removed during processing have been added back in. And today folic acid (folate) is being added as well. A particular advantage to whole-wheat bread, however, is that it includes the germ, which is rich in vitamin E, one of the major antioxidants.

Pasta

Most pastas are made from durum wheat flour and water. They are a modest source of protein for vegetarians, particularly when eaten with legumes. Pastas are also low in calories and are therefore ideal for a weight-control program, as long as creamy sauces are not used with them.

For people who cannot eat pasta because of an intolerance for gluten, a few brands are made with Jerusalem artichokes. (See pages 141–142 for more information on a gluten-free diet plan.)

STARCHES FROM VEGETABLES

It is in the roots and tubers of plants where much of their energy is stored, and thus the ones we eat supply a good amount of starch. The starchy vegetables include Jerusalem artichokes, potatoes, and cassava.

Potatoes

As well as being a rich source of starch, potatoes provide fiber. Most of it is in the skin, so you must eat the skin to get the full cholesterol-lowering effect. Potatoes are a valuable source of protein if eaten in large quantities and are low in fat, but they can

BEST BREAD

Because white breads are made with enriched flour, there is little difference between whole-wheat and white bread except in the fiber. Added seeds and grains will increase fiber and protein.

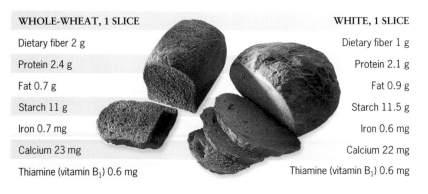

WHOLE-WHEAT, 1 SLICE	WHITE, 1 SLICE
Dietary fiber 2 g	Dietary fiber 1 g
Protein 2.4 g	Protein 2.1 g
Fat 0.7 g	Fat 0.9 g
Starch 11 g	Starch 11.5 g
Iron 0.7 mg	Iron 0.6 mg
Calcium 23 mg	Calcium 22 mg
Thiamine (vitamin B$_1$) 0.6 mg	Thiamine (vitamin B$_1$) 0.6 mg

absorb a large amount of fat during some cooking methods, especially deep frying.

Potatoes supply a good amount of vitamin C in a diet if eaten often, but like other vegetables, they lose their vitamin C content with age and cooking; much of it is lost to the cooking water when potatoes are boiled. Potatoes also contain useful amounts of iron, potassium, zinc, and the B vitamins, which are concentrated in and beneath the skin. Most of the fiber is located there too, so eating the skin as well as the flesh provides the most benefit.

Do not buy potatoes that have green spots or sprouts. The sprouts indicate that the tubers are old, and the green color is a toxic substance called solanine. If your potatoes have turned green since you bought them, peel and cook them thoroughly. Stored in a cool, dark place (but not in the refrigerator, where their starch turns to sugar), potatoes will keep for up to two months.

Cassava

Cassava, also called yuca, is the swollen root of a tropical plant that looks like a long potato. It is rich in starch and contains a significant amount of vitamin C. Cassava has a high cyanide content, which is concentrated in the peel. The toxic effects are reduced by peeling and boiling.

Boiled cassava develops a soft, floury texture and tastes similar to a potato. Cassava roots are often fried; they can also be roasted or baked, just like the potato. Tapioca, used to thicken puddings, is made from cassava.

Sweet potato

The sweet potato is rich in starch and has a moderately good content of protein and potassium. It has more calcium and vitamin C than a regular potato and is an outstanding source of beta carotene. Like the white potato, the sweet potato can be baked, boiled (preferably whole to avoid becoming mushy), mashed, steamed, or fried, and added to stews and casseroles. With added sugar, spices, and eggs, it also makes a fine pudding or a filling for a dessert pie.

Yam

The true yam is a tuber grown in tropical areas, particularly Africa. It is rich in starch and is a good source of potassium but is low in vitamins; it has virtually no vitamin A. This root can be fried, baked, or boiled and

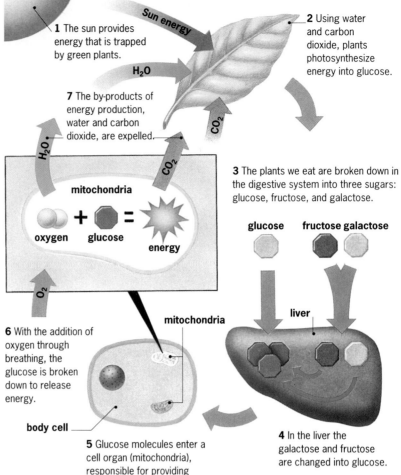

1 The sun provides energy that is trapped by green plants.

Sun energy

2 Using water and carbon dioxide, plants photosynthesize energy into glucose.

H_2O

7 The by-products of energy production, water and carbon dioxide, are expelled.

H_2O

CO_2

CO_2

3 The plants we eat are broken down in the digestive system into three sugars: glucose, fructose, and galactose.

mitochondria

oxygen + glucose = energy

glucose   fructose galactose

liver

O_2

6 With the addition of oxygen through breathing, the glucose is broken down to release energy.

mitochondria

body cell

5 Glucose molecules enter a cell organ (mitochondria), responsible for providing energy for the cell.

4 In the liver the galactose and fructose are changed into glucose.

included in a variety of savory dishes. It is usually available only in Hispanic markets.

The yam most familiar to North Americans and found typically in supermarkets is a relative of the sweet potato and has the same characteristics and nutrients.

Plantain

Plantain, a fruit grown in tropical countries, is related to the banana. However, it contains more starch, beta carotene, and potassium than the banana and is high in fiber. It is normally prepared as a savory dish (often fried) and sometimes pground to form flour or meal. Some cooks boil or steam it, then mash it and serve it with meat.

Jerusalem artichoke

Also known as the sunchoke, this tuber is related to the sunflower and is very high in iron and fiber. It can be eaten raw or cooked (boiled, baked, sautéed, steamed, or stir-fried) and is best consumed with its skin on because the nutrients are concentrated there.

STARCH INTO ENERGY
Plants take energy from the sun and create starches, which in turn can be transformed into energy in the body and used to fuel the body's systems.

LEGUMES

One of the world's oldest food crops, legumes contain more protein than any other plant food. They are also high in fiber, the B vitamins, iron, and potassium and low in fat.

BEANS AND SOLUBLE FIBER
Soluble fiber, found in such legumes as lentils, chickpeas (also called garbanzo beans), red kidney beans, and adzuki (also called azuki) beans, shown below, is broken down in the large intestine. It helps reduce the level of LDLs ("bad cholesterol) in the blood.

Thousands of legumes are cultivated around the world. They vary greatly but have two traits in common: all produce seed-bearing pods and their roots replenish the soil with nitrogen, a nutrient depleted by other food crops, especially grains. Just the seeds of some legumes are eaten. Examples are lima, kidney, fava, and pinto beans, lentils, and chickpeas. With other legumes, such as snowpeas and green beans, both the pod and its contents are eaten.

With a few exceptions—green peas, fava beans, lima beans, cranberry beans, and soybeans—the seeds of legumes are dried before cooking. This concentrates their nutrients and boosts their status of "superfood." They are good sources of starch, protein, B vitamins, iron, potassium, zinc, and other essential minerals.

Legumes also provide a useful amount of soluble fiber, which is especially important to people with diabetes because it slows absorption of sugar from the small intestine into the bloodstream after meals, thus reducing the need for insulin. Also, several studies have suggested that soluble fiber reduces cholesterol levels overall and helps raise levels of HDLs ("good" cholesterol).

The protein in legumes, unlike that in fish, meat, eggs, and dairy products, is not complete; it does not provide all the amino acids the body needs for growth and tissue repair. To obtain the full benefit of their protein, legumes should be combined with a grain such as rice, barley, or corn in the same meal or another meal on the same day. The iron in legumes is better absorbed if a food containing vitamin C is consumed along with it. This could be a glass of orange juice or tomatoes added to the cooking water.

OLIGOSACCHARIDES

Peas and beans, as well as leeks, artichokes, onions, garlic, cabbage, apples, and some cereals, contain oligosaccharides. These are complex sugars that are not digested in the stomach and small intestine as other carbohydrates are. Instead, they pass through the digestive system to the large intestine, where there is a rich culture of bacteria that breaks them down into substances called short-chain fatty acids and the gases hydrogen and carbon dioxide. These are the source of the intestinal gas that many people experience after eating beans.

Allthough the side effects of oligosaccharides are unpleasant, they may have some benefits. Research studies on animals indicate that a culture of good bacteria in the large bowel helps prevent cancer there and lowers blood cholesterol levels. Oligosaccharides encourage beneficial bacteria to grow in the large bowel.

SOYBEANS

Soybeans stand out among legumes because they have a few special characteristics. First, they have the highest protein content of all legumes—about 40 percent of the dry weight is protein. Moreover, soy protein is of better quality than that of other beans because it has more of the essential amino acids. Soybeans also contain more calcium than other legumes, as well as phytoestrogen, the less potent plant equivalent of the female hormone estrogen. For this reason soybeans and soy products are believed to help reduce the risk of certain types of breast cancer (see page 40). On the down side, they are much higher in fat than other legumes, although it is an unsaturated type.

Soybeans were originally grown as an oil seed crop, but the residue left after the oil was extracted became equally valued as an excellent source of high-quality protein. This residue is widely used to make tofu, a white curd made from soybean milk (soybeans that have been soaked, puréed, cooked, and coagulated with calcium sulfate).

Soy protein can be found in such forms as tofu, tempeh, soy milk, and textured vegetable protein, available in supermarkets and health food stores. Unfortunately, soy sauce does not have the same beneficial effect.

BEAN SPROUTS

Many kinds of bean sprouts are available in health food stores and supermarkets today, including mung bean, lentil, chickpea, alfalfa, and soybean. All can be eaten raw except soybean sprouts, which contain a toxin that is destroyed by cooking.

Nutritional content varies. A cupful of the familiar mung bean sprouts, often used in Chinese stir-fries, has a generous amount of folate and other B vitamins, plus vitamin C. It would take five cups of alfalfa sprouts to provide a similiar amount. Because they are low in calories, all sprouts are a good snack for a weight-control program.

When buying bean sprouts, look for ones that are crisp and slightly dry. They should not be wet, soft, or brown around the edges.

LEGUMES WITH EDIBLE PODS

Beans and peas with edible pods, which are picked at a less mature stage than other legumes, include green (or snap) beans, wax beans, snowpeas, and sugar snap peas. These contain much smaller amounts of protein, carbohydrate, fiber, and iron than mature, dried legumes, but are moderate sources of vitamin C and beta carotene. To retain these nutrients, it is best to cook them as briefly and in as little water as possible. They will also retain their appealing green color with this treatment. Sugar snaps and snowpeas are good, too, when stir-fried for a couple of minutes. Green beans need to cook for at least 6 to 8 minutes.

COOKING DRIED LEGUMES

Before cooking dried legumes, always rinse them and pick them over. With the exception of lentils and split peas, they also need to be soaked before cooking. There are two ways to do this. The first, the "long-soak method," is to put them in a large bowl, add enough cold water to cover them by 2 inches, and soak for 4 to 8 hours. The second, called "quick soaking," is to put them in a large saucepan, cover them with ample cold water, bring them to a boil, then turn off the heat and let them stand for 1 hour. The soaking water should be discarded and the beans rinsed thoroughly. Some experts recommend changing the water a few times during the soaking process; this seems to lessen the gas-forming potential

Cook beans gently over low heat. You can include flavoring ingredients, such as onions, garlic, and herbs while they cook, but don't add salt until the last minute because salt toughens beans. Cooking time will vary according to the type of bean and how old they are; freshly dried beans will cook more quickly. Lentils and split peas usually cook in about 45 minutes, all other types in 1 to 2 hours.

Because canned beans usually contain a great deal of salt, it is a good idea to rinse them thoroughly before adding them to soups, casseroles, salads, and other dishes.

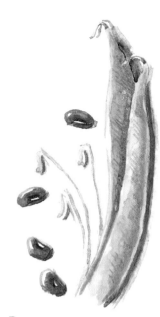

BEAN BENEFITS
Low in calories and fat, beans, peas, and other legumes are relatively high in protein, iron, fiber, and the B vitamins.

NUTRIENT CONTENT OF VARIOUS LEGUMES

The figures below are for a ½-cup serving (3–4 ounces) of cooked dried beans. Soybeans are the highest in protein, iron, and fat, although the fat is unsaturated. Those with the lowest fat content are lentils and kidney beans.

TYPE OF BEAN	CALORIES	PROTEIN (g)	FAT (g)	FIBER (g)	IRON (mg)
Soybean	170	15	7.5	3	4.5
Chickpea	164	8	3	3.1	3.0
Lentil	116	9	0.5	5.0	3.3
Red kidney	127	9	0.5	7.4	2.7

NUTS AND SEEDS

Cultivated for more than 10,000 years, nuts and seeds are valuable sources of many essential nutrients and should be included on your superfood list.

Because they are packed with the nutrients to grow a new plant, nuts and seeds are nutritional powerhouses. They are rich in potassium and vitamin E— a powerful antioxidant that helps protect the body's cells from the damaging effects of free radicals (see page 50) and also protect against heart disease. Most are also relatively high in iron, magnesium, calcium, and zinc. Some nuts are good sources of the B vitamins except B$_{12}$, and a few provide useful amounts of dietary fiber.

Nuts and seeds are especially important in vegetarian diets because they are a relatively concentrated source of protein. However, the protein is not complete unless combined with grains because it is deficient in the amino acid lysine.

A significant fact about nuts and seeds is that they are high in fat, with each type containing varying proportions of saturated and unsaturated forms but mostly unsaturated. On the plus side, their fat includes the polyunsaturated linoleic acid, an essential

fatty acid that the body cannot function normally without. On the minus side, their fat content means that they are high in calories; also, they tend to go rancid if kept for any length of time.

ALMONDS

Much of the fat in almonds is monounsaturated. Monounsaturated fat is effective at lowering LDLs when consumed in place of saturated fat. Almonds and hazelnuts (also known as filberts) are also high in calcium.

Avoid almonds that have not matured fully; they contain compounds that produce the poisonous gas hydrogen cyanide.

BRAZIL NUTS

Compared to other nuts, Brazils contain a large amount of saturated fat and should therefore be eaten in small amounts only. However, they are a good source of the antioxidant mineral selenium, which fights cancer, and they have been linked with the prevention of stomach cancer.

SUNFLOWER SEEDS

Although most nuts and seeds have nutritional benefits, sunflower seeds are particularly rich in healthy nutrients. The following amounts are per 25 grams.

Energy	142 kcal	Protein	5.6 g
Dietary fiber	1.4 g	Calcium	29.5 mg
		Potassium	173.5 mg
		Iron	1.7 mg
		Zinc	1.25 mg
		Vitamin E	9.5 mg
		B vitamins	2 mg
		Fat	12.6 g

THE BEST OF NUTS AND SEEDS
Nuts and seeds contain useful amounts of protein, vitamin E, B vitamins, dietary fiber, potassium, iron, zinc, and calcium. Sunflower seeds (separate wedge below) are particularly rich in these nutrients.

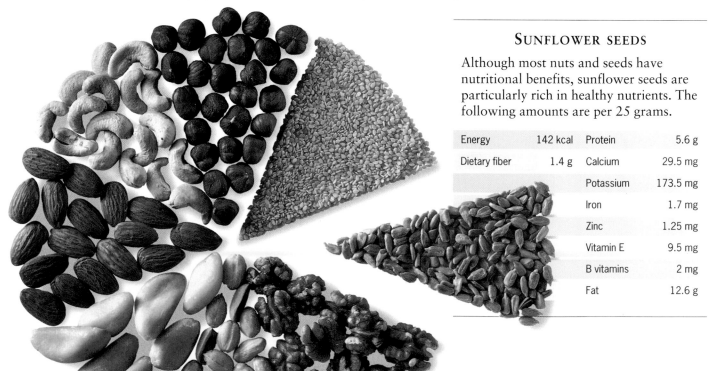

NUTRIENT CONTENT OF VARIOUS NUTS AND SEEDS

1 OZ SERVING	CALORIES	PROTEIN (g)	FAT (g)	FIBER (g)	IRON (mg)	ZINC (mg)	VITAMIN E (mg)
Almonds	170	5.3	15.4	1.9	1.3	0.8	6.0
Brazil nuts	185	4.1	19	1.1	1.0	1.0	1.8
Cashew nuts	159	5.1	13.0	0.8	1.5	1.4	0.4
Hazelnuts	85	3.5	18.6	1.6	0.8	0.5	6.3
Peanuts, roasted	156	7.2	13.3	1.5	0.6	0.7	0.2
Sesame seeds	150	4.5	14.5	2.0	2.5	1.3	0.8
Pumpkin seeds	156	8.2	13.2	1.8	3.8	1.9	0.25
Walnuts (English)	185	4.2	18.1	0.9	0.9	0.6	1.0

CASHEW NUTS

Cashews contain a higher amount of saturated fat than hazelnuts, walnuts, and almonds. However, they are a good source of phosphorous and potassium.

CHESTNUTS

The uniqueness of chestnuts is that they are low in fat and calories. One ounce of chestnuts contains 0.2 grams of fat and 70 calories, compared with 13 grams of fat and 159 calories for cashews. They are also good sources of several important nutrients, including vitamins B_6, C, and folate.

PEANUTS

Peanuts are not actually nuts but the seeds of a leguminous plant that are roasted and eaten out of hand like nuts. Peanut butter is a paste of ground roasted peanuts, often mixed with salt, sweeteners, and stabilizers. Peanuts contain more protein than other nuts and a mixture of unsaturated fat with a small amount of saturates. They are good sources of fiber, iron, and B vitamins.

One problem with peanuts is that they are susceptible to a toxic mold called aflatoxin, which is a carcinogen. It's best to buy peanuts from sources that have been government inspected. Also, some people are allergic to them and can have severe reactions.

WALNUTS

One study on walnuts found a 10 percent reduction in blood cholesterol levels in men who were put on a low-fat diet that was supplemented with 80 grams of walnuts daily. While this research looks promising, more evidence is required before strong conclusions can be drawn. Most of the fat in walnuts is polyunsaturated; they are a particularly good source of linoleic fatty acid.

PUMPKIN SEEDS

Pumpkin seeds are very high in phosphorous and potassium. They also provide measurable amounts of iron and calcium, and because of their zinc content, naturopaths recommend that men with prostate problems eat plenty of them.

SUNFLOWER SEEDS

The majority of fat in sunflower seeds is polyunsaturated, which raises levels of HDLs ("good" cholesterol). Sunflower seed oil is the basis of some cooking oils.

SESAME SEEDS

Sesame seeds contain roughly equal amounts of monounsaturated and polyunsaturated fats and a much smaller amount of saturates. They are a reasonable source of iron and calcium and so are particularly useful for vegans. The ground seeds are combined with mashed chickpeas in the popular dish tahini.

BUYING AND STORING GUIDE

Nuts should be crisp and blemish-free. It is best to buy nuts and seeds as you need them because they have a high fat content and can go rancid fairly quickly. If you must keep them for a while, store them in the freezer or refrigerator.

NUTTY IDEAS

Nuts can be used in a variety of dishes to add a crunchy texture. Below are a few ideas.

▶ *Scatter pine nuts, cashews, or sesame seeds over green salads. For a unique flavor, roast pine nuts in a little soy sauce first.*

▶ *When making a stir-fry, add cashews or sesame seeds just before serving.*

▶ *Add toasted walnuts and sesame seeds or caraway seeds to shredded and boiled green cabbage.*

▶ *Add flavor to baked potatoes with a sprinkling of caraway seeds.*

▶ *Use nuts to garnish dishes. Toasted almonds sprinkled over casseroles, vegetables, and steamed rice add crunchy texture as well as nutrients.*

▶ *Sprinkle chopped nuts over yogurt or fruit, add them to muffins and other breads, or use them to decorate cakes.*

FISH, SHELLFISH, AND SEAWEED

Valuable sources of protein as well as several vitamins and minerals, fish and shellfish have fewer calories and less fat than comparable portions of meat.

Omega-3 during pregnancy and breast-feeding
One of the omega-3 fatty acids in fish, docosahexaenoic acid (DHA), is particularly important during pregnancy and breast-feeding. DHA is required for the development of the fetal brain and eye, and limited clinical research to date suggests that insufficient DHA can impair learning ability and eyesight.

FISH
Low in saturated fat, fish are excellent sources of protein, phosphorous, selenium, zinc, iodine, magnesium, iron, and omega-3 fatty acids.

Because it is generally low in fat but high in complete protein and essential vitamins and minerals, seafood has long played an important part in healthy eating. Because of their omega-3 fatty acids, fish, especially cold-water types, are considered a healthy alternative to red meat for everyone, but especially those who have hypertension, high cholesterol levels, and heart disease. The American Heart Association (AHA) recommends three or more servings of fish a week to obtain the benefits.

OILY FISH

The fat in oily, or cold-water, fish—which include bluefish, anchovies, haddock, mackerel, pompano, salmon, fresh sardines, swordfish, shad, and albacore tuna—is spread throughout the body. Although the total fat in these fish can be comparable to that of lean beef, most of it is unsaturated and rich in omega-3 fatty acids, which have special benefits that lower the risk of heart attack. They raise levels of HDLs ("good" cholesterol) in the blood, lower LDLs ("bad" cholesterol), and make the blood less sticky or likely to clot. Some studies suggest that these benefits of omega-3 fatty acids may be useful in preventing gallstones as well. Fat and cholesterol are involved in the formation of gallstones.

Yet another benefit for oily fish has been uncovered in studies concerning asthma. Omega-3 fatty acids help reduce inflammation in the lungs and may actually prevent the onset of asthma in children who are served fish often.

Fish oil supplements show promise in bringing relief from psoriasis and the symptoms of rheumatoid arthritis. However, there is a danger in taking these supplements, especially in combination with aspirin or another blood-thinning agent. Their contents are not regulated for safety; most are high in calories and cholesterol, and many also contain vitamins A and D, which are toxic in large doses. You should use a supplement only if your doctor prescribes a particular brand and monitors your health.

LEAN FISH

Much of the fat in lean, or white, fish is stored in the liver, so that the flesh of these species contain less than half the fat of oily fish. The livers of cod and halibut are among the highest natural sources of vitamins A and D; hence the widespread use, at one time, of cod liver oil as a supplement.

Typical examples of white fish are flounder, cod, monkfish, snapper, and tilefish.

A concern with fish today is contamination from polluted waters. Most bacteria in fish are killed by freezing. Contaminants from industrial or agricultural runoff can only be avoided. Become informed about problem waters and buy from a reliable fishmonger who can tell you the source of the catch. Farmed fish are usually safe.

Buying and storing guide
Fresh fish should have a shiny, moist skin and firm flesh. The eyes should be clear, bright, and not appear sunken. Before storing in the refrigerator, unwrap the fish, place it on a dish, and cover it.

Cooking tips
Any cooking method that requires little or no oil is preferable, such as broiling under a medium heat. Microwaving works well too, and poaching in water, low-fat milk, or fish stock maintains the flavor without adding too much fat to the dish. Steaming, poaching, and baking are particularly good because they keep the succulent flesh of the fish flavorful and moist.

SHELLFISH
There are two main types of shellfish: crustaceans and mollusks. Crustaceans have legs with partly jointed outer shells; they include crabs, lobsters, and shrimp. Mollusks have hard outer shells and no legs. Some, such as oysters, scallops, abalone, and mussels, have hinged shells. Snails have shells in one piece.

Oysters and clams are often eaten raw. Any shellfish to be eaten raw must come from a clean source. If gathered near outlets of urban sewage, they can harbor bacteria, particularly salmonella, and hepatitis.

Shellfish are one of the best dietary sources of iodine, which assists in the formation of thyroid hormones, which control development and growth and aid in the production of energy inside the body's cells.

Some people avoid shellfish because they contain cholesterol. However, shellfish are relatively low in saturated fat, and the saturated fat in food has a greater impact on blood cholesterol levels than the cholesterol content. Moreover, some types are relatively low in cholesterol, having about the same amount per ounce as chicken breasts.

Buying and storing guide
When buying shellfish, make sure that the shells are not cracked or broken; mussel and oyster shells should be tightly shut. A good-quality mussel is one that is partly open but that closes tightly when tapped. Lobsters, crabs, and shrimp should all have a strong color, and there would be no unpleasant smell from the flesh or the shell. Like all seafood, shellfish should smell fresh and slightly of the sea. Most are highly perishable and are best used immediately.

SEAWEED
Seaweed is low in fat and has a high mineral content, including iodine, iron, copper, magnesium, calcium, and potassium. Although it contains only a little protein, seaweed offers varying amounts of B vitamins and the antioxidant beta-carotene. It is also, however, high in sodium.

Certain omega-3 fatty acids are present in some species of seaweed, and they have fair amounts of vitamin B_{12}. This makes seaweed a good choice for vegetarians, especially for vegans, who eat no animal products.

Agar and alginic acid are seaweed derivatives that are added to foods like jellies to set them or yogurts to thicken them. Agar-agar is available in some health food and Asian stores as a vegetarian alternative to gelatin, derived from calves feet.

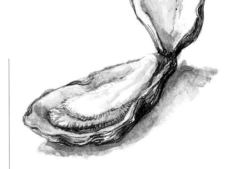

Are oysters an aphrodisiac?
For centuries oysters have been touted as aphrodisiacs. While there is no scientific evidence that oysters improve sexual drive or enhance sexual performance, the oyster may have gained its reputation because of its high zinc content. Zinc is essential for the normal and healthy functioning of the reproductive system in both men and women.

SHELLFISH
The main nutrients provided by shellfish are protein, B vitamins, zinc, calcium, copper, selenium, potassium, and iodine.

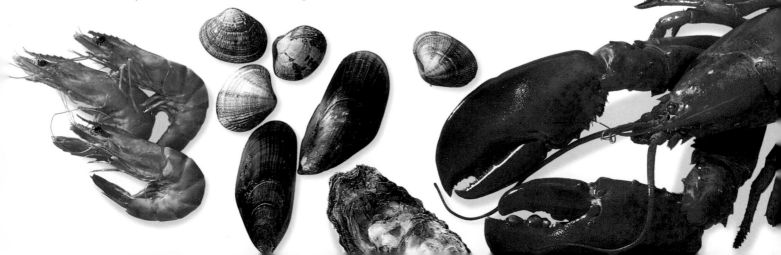

MEAT AND EGGS

While warnings about the negative aspects of too much meat or too many eggs should be heeded, when eaten in moderation, both are excellent sources of essential nutrients.

In recent years meat and eggs have had a fair amount of bad press because of their cholesterol and saturated fat content and hence their link to heart disease and certain types of cancer. However, in moderation, meat and eggs play an important part in a healthy, balanced diet.

MEAT

Red meat—beef, veal, lamb, and pork—and poultry—chicken, turkey, duck, goose, and Cornish hens—earn a "superfood" title because they provide high-quality protein, which contains all the essential amino acids needed by the body to build and repair tissues. Meat is also an excellent source of B vitamins, necessary for many bodily processes, particularly metabolism.

Vitamin B_{12}, used in producing red blood cells, is present mainly in animal foods (and to some extent in fermented products and seaweed). A 4-ounce serving of meat provides 100 percent of the Recommended Dietary Allowance (RDA) of B_{12}.

Meat and important minerals

Red meat is a good source of potassium, as well as zinc and other trace elements, such as copper, manganese, and selenium, an antioxidant. In fact, animal feed in some regions is fortified with selenium. Poultry, particularly turkey and duck, is also an excellent source of zinc and potassium.

Meat and poultry are also the most useful sources of iron, needed for the formation of healthy red blood cells; a low intake of iron is the most common dietary cause of anemia. Some people are more vulnerable to iron deficiency than others. They include menstruating women, who lose iron in blood flow every month; elderly people, some of whom may have poor appetites and poor nutrient absorption; and toddlers, who are growing rapidly and using more energy.

Iron absorption

It is not just the amount of iron in food that is important, but how well it is absorbed by the body from various food sources. Heme iron, the kind present in meat, is more easily absorbed than the nonheme iron found in plants. Absorption from nonheme iron is much less reliable and can be affected by other dietary components. For example, milk, tea, coffee, and substances called phytates in raw bran from cereals reduce iron absorption. However, vitamin C aids the absorption of iron from nonheme sources.

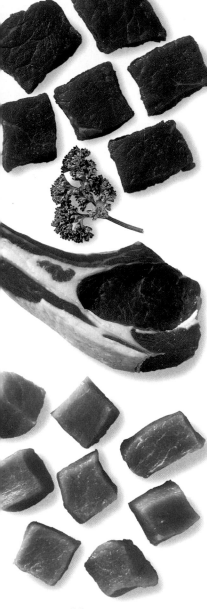

MEAT MATTERS
Beef, lamb, and pork can be trimmed to remove as much fat as possible.

NUTRIENT CONTENT OF VARIOUS MEATS

Many people shy away from red meat because they fear increased cholesterol levels from its saturated fat; indeed, even very lean meat contains some. Meat, however, is an important source of protein, B vitamins, and minerals such as iron.

3½ OZ SERVING	FAT (g)	SATURATED FAT (g)	PROTEIN (g)	NIACIN (mg)	IRON (mg)
Beef round	2.7	1	29.2	3.76	1.3
Leg of lamb	4.7	2.1	28.3	6.36	2
Leg of pork	2	0.6–0.8	31	4.92	0.9

Meat and fat

More than 60 percent of the calories in red meat come from fat (there is less in the light meat of turkey and chicken), and much of this fat is saturated. The meat with the highest fat content is labeled "prime." This is the type that hasmarbling—fat is distributed throughout the meat, which makes it juicier, more tender, and also more expensive. Meat with the next highest amount of fat is called "choice"; the type with the lowest is termed "select." In addition to these labels, fat in meat is determined by the part of the animal that it comes from. The round is one of the leaner parts.

Today's figures on fat in meat represent an improvement. Over the past 20 years, the fat content has been reduced to meet consumer demands. A number of processes have contributed to this, including selective breeding and changes in animal feed and butchery techniques. Many cuts of beef, lamb, and pork now contain a fat level similar to that of chicken, and much of it is unsaturated rather than saturated (see page 79).

Buying and storing guide

When buying meats, look for even-colored flesh and firm fat; avoid any cuts that appear wet, greenish gray, or have an off smell. Store whole meats, loosely covered, in the coldest part of the refrigerator for no more than five days. Use ground meat immediately.

EGGS

Eggs are a nearly perfect food: They are low-cost providers of complete protein and a rich storehouse of nutrients, including vitamins A, D, E, and B_{12} plus iron, zinc, and other minerals. The amount of vitamin B_{12} in one large egg is one-fourth the daily

---

WARNING

A potentially deadly type of E. coli *infection has been traced to contaminated beef. In most people it causes mild to severe diarrhea, but in those with weak immune systems—young children or the elderly, for example— these bacteria can bring on a disorder that destroys red blood cells and causes kidney failure. Such infections can be prevented by cooking beef, especially hamburger, until well done.*

WHAT'S IN AN EGG?

The nutritional value of an egg is far from evenly split between yolk and white; all the cholesterol and fat in an egg is in the yolk.

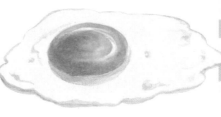

	YOLK	WHITE
Fat	5 g	0
Cholesterol	212 mg	0
Protein	3 g	4 g
Vitamin A	97 mg	0
Vitamin B_{12}	.44 mcg	.06 mcg
Potassium	16 mg	48 mg
Phosphorus	81 mg	4 mg
Sodium	9 mg	48 mg

---

requirement for an adult, so eggs are a particularly good food for vegetarians. Eggs also contain choline, important for fat and cholesterol metabolism and healthy cell membranes. To top things off, eggs are also low in calories; one large egg has only 75.

In the yolk reside all of the egg's fat-soluble vitamins, A, D, and E, the fat, and the cholesterol. It is because of the cholesterol content that some people avoid eggs. However, it is generally not the cholesterol in food that increases blood cholesterol but the amount of saturated fat. The fat in egg yolks (5 to 6 grams) is made up mainly of the beneficial monounsaturated fatty acids; only 2 grams are saturated.

To keep cholesterol intake to 300 milligrams per day, the American Heart Association recommends that adults eat no more than four egg yolks per week, including the ones in baked goods. Whites can be eaten in unlimited quantities and, in fact, can be substituted for whole eggs (two whites for each whole egg) in many recipes.

Commerical egg substitutes are available in frozen, refrigerated, and powdered forms. They consist largely of egg whites plus some food coloring and vegetable oil. Although most contain little or no cholesterol, many have about the same fat content as a whole egg. These products can be used to replace eggs in recipes and to make scrambled eggs.

Buying and storing guide

Always check the use-by date on eggs and make sure they are not cracked. Store eggs in their carton in the refrigerator. To check if an egg is fresh, put it in a bowl of water. If it sinks it is fine; if it floats, throw it away. An old egg floats because bacteria in the egg create gases that make it buoyant.

Cooking eggs for health

Eggs (and poultry) occasionally harbor salmonella bacteria. Although the risk of encountering salmonella is fairly low, it's best not to eat raw or partly cooked eggs. Both the yolk and white should be firm. People at high risk, such as pregnant women, the elderly, young children, and anyone with lowered immunity, should be especially careful.

MILK AND OTHER DAIRY FOODS

Major sources of calcium, which is essential for healthy bones and teeth and various bodily functions, milk and dairy foods also contain other important nutrients.

DAIRY DELIGHTS
Milk, yogurt, and cheese, although sometimes high in fat, also offer protein, calcium, and other essential elements in a healthy diet.

The nutrients provided by milk and other dairy products include protein, calcium, vitamin B_{12}, vitamins A and D, and phosphorus. (Note that vitamin B_{12} is destroyed when milk is boiled.) A major drawback of whole milk and products made from it is the high fat content, most of which is saturated, but a wide selection of low-fat and nonfat products is now available.

PROTECTIVE PROPERTIES

It is the high content of calcium in milk and dairy foods that qualifies them as superfoods. Calcium is associated with protection from a number of disorders, including osteoporosis (see page 46), high blood pressure, and possibly colon cancer. Phosphorus, another nutrient present in useful amounts in milk, is also essential for bone health.

Calcium makes up about 2 percent of your total body weight, and most of it (approximately 99 percent) is found in the bones and teeth. Calcium also has a major role in regulating metabolic processes, such as blood clotting and muscular contractions. An adequate dietary intake of calcium throughout life is therefore vital.

During childhood and early adulthood, bones are continually accumulating calcium in large amounts. Between ages 18 and 30, bones are no longer actually growing, but they continue to thicken and increase in density and strength until what is known as peak bone mass is reached. After this pinnacle is achieved, there is a gradual age-related loss of bone density in both men and women. The loss accelerates in women for 5 to 10 years after menopause, making them particularly susceptible to bone problems such as osteoporosis.

It seems increasingly clear that it is possible to prevent osteoporosis from developing or worsening if individuals make sure that they eat enough calcium-rich foods through-

ACHIEVING OPTIMAL DIETARY CALCIUM INTAKE

Although small amounts of calcium can be found in nondairy foods such as legumes, broccoli, the soft bones of canned fish, and dried fruit, it is not as easily absorbed as that in dairy foods. Dairy foods also contain phosphorus, magnesium, vitamin D, and riboflavin—essential nutrients for bone health. For a daily calcium intake of about 1,000 mg, choose two to three servings of dairy products, as shown below.

Milk 240 ml (8 ounces)			**Cheese 50 g (2 oz)**		**Nonfat cottage cheese 150 g (6 oz)**	**Low-fat yogurt 150 g (8 oz)**
Nonfat	1 percent	Whole	Cheddar	Swiss		
296 mg.	292mg	288 mg	426 mg	524 mg	156 mg	270 mg

out life; do regular weight-bearing exercise, such as walking and aerobics; do not smoke or consume excessive amounts of alcohol; and (for women) have hormone replacement therapy after menopause.

How much calcium do you need?

To keep a healthy reserve of calcium in the body, a calcium-rich diet is vital. Calcium requirements vary according to age and gender. Children should have 800 to 1,200 milligrams per day. Adolescent girls need a minimum of 1,200 mg per day, while adolescent boys need about 1,500 mg. Pregnant women require 1,200 to 1,500 mg. Women and men past 50 should have at least 1,000 mg a day, while menopausal women not on hormone replacement therapy need 1,500 mg. Men and women over 65 years should aim for at least 1,500 mg per day.

Surplus calcium is usually excreted, but taking too much can block absorption of iron and zinc, especially if they come from supplements. Check with your doctor.

People who have trouble digesting cow's milk because of lactose intolerance may find that they have no problem with yogurt, which contains less lactose. Alternatively, they can try goat's milk or soy milk that is fortified with the nutrients that cow's milk contains. Children who cannot drink cow's milk will usually need a calcium supplement.

YOGURT AND HEALTH

Yogurt is pasteurized milk to which live cultures of the bacteria *Lactobacillus bulgaricus* and *Streptococcus thermophilus* have been added. They often contain *Bifobacteri bifidum* and *L. acidophilus* as well. These convert lactose, or milk sugar, to lactic acid, thus curdling the milk. The end product has the same protein, vitamin, and mineral content of the milk with which it was made. Sometimes extra milk solids; fruit, fruit juice, or other flavorings; sugar or nonsugar sweetener; and modified cornstarch, pectin, and/or gelatin have been added.

A big advantage of yogurt is that it is more easily digested than milk and can be tolerated by many people who are intolerant to lactose. Recently there has been particular interest in the role of special microorganisms in yogurt and the health benefits these confer. Most of yogurt's active bacteria are destroyed during digestion and so offer no additional benefits to the body.

Some types of bacteria, namely *L. acidophilus* and *B. bifidum,* are able to survive the digestive process and remain active in the large intestine. These "good" bacteria prevent harmful organisms from growing there. Research studies with animals suggest that the good bacteria may stimulate the immune system, lower cholesterol levels, and reduce the risk of colon cancer. So far, the only proven benefit is that *L. acidophilus* reduces the incidence of vaginal yeast infections.

Yogurt cheese, plain yogurt from which the whey has been drained, can be spread on bread like cream cheese or used as a low-fat alternative to whipped cream. To make it, pour yogurt into a strainer lined with cheesecloth, set the strainer over a glass bowl, cover, and refrigerate for a day or two.

OTHER DAIRY PRODUCTS

Cheeses have the nutritional benefits of milk, but most are also high in saturated fats and should be eaten in moderation. The cheeses highest in fat include Cheddar, Parmesan, Stilton, Brie, and Camembert. Ricotta and cottage cheese have lower fat contents.

Buttermilk, which contains bacteria cultures, is very low in fat, with a similar nutritional content to that of skim milk. Creams are very high in saturated fat and should be eaten sparingly. However, sour cream is now available in reduced-fat and nonfat versions.

GUIDE TO CHOOSING YOGURT

Commercial yogurts range from plain versions to creamy types with additives, such as fruit, fruit juice, sugar or nonsugar sweetener, and gelatin. Fat content varies.

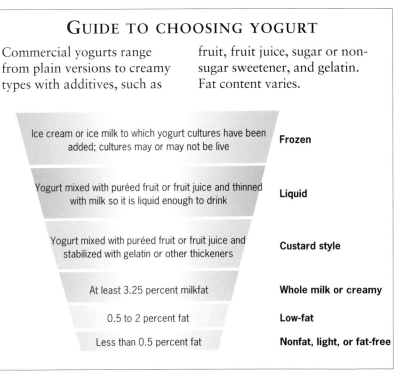

Ice cream or ice milk to which yogurt cultures have been added; cultures may or may not be live	**Frozen**
Yogurt mixed with puréed fruit or fruit juice and thinned with milk so it is liquid enough to drink	**Liquid**
Yogurt mixed with puréed fruit or fruit juice and stabilized with gelatin or other thickeners	**Custard style**
At least 3.25 percent milkfat	**Whole milk or creamy**
0.5 to 2 percent fat	**Low-fat**
Less than 0.5 percent fat	**Nonfat, light, or fat-free**

FATS

Small amounts of fat in the diet are essential for good health: they supply essential fatty acids, circulate the fat soluble vitamins, make food more palatable, and provide energy.

How much fat should you have?

The amount of fat you should consume is related to your calorie requirements. These vary according to gender, age, physical activity, and body weight. In general, however, fat calories should be no more than 30 percent of the daily total, and 10 percent or less should saturated.

Fats serve a number of important functions in the human body. The kind that comes from your food—dietary fat—supplies energy in the form of calories, aids in the absorption of the fat-soluble vitamins, A, D, E, and K, provides essential fatty acids that the body cannot function normally without, and makes food more palatable. Body fat, stored when caloric intake exceeds what the body needs at the moment, serves as an energy reserve, helps keep the body warm, and cushions the internal organs.

TYPES OF FAT

There are three types of fat—polyunsaturated, monounsaturated, and saturated—and they differ in chemical structure and function. It is well known that saturated fats, the type that is prevalent in the Western diet, can damage the body by raising the levels of triglycerides that lay down fatty plaques to clog arteries. Poly- and monounsaturated fats can help undo some of the damage caused by saturated fats.

Polyunsaturated fats

Polyunsatuarated fats, abundant in vegetable oils, nuts, seeds, and oily fish, are always in a liquid state unless hydrogen has been added by the process known as hydrogenation. (Margarine is a product of hydrogenation.) Two forms of polyunsaturated fat, linoleic acid and linolenic acid, are classified as essential fatty acids because the body needs them to function normally.

Research studies have shown that most polyunsaturated fats, when substituted for saturated ones in the diet, effectively reduce the LDLs ("bad" cholesterol), associated with heart disease and stroke, without lowering HDLs ("good" cholesterol).

The type of polyunsaturated fats known as omega-3 fatty acids are especially important in preventing blood clots and lowering blood cholesterol levels. These fats also help relieve psoriasis and arthritis in some people, probably by reducing the production of prostaglandins, which contribute to inflammation. They appear to play a role as well

---

DIETARY SOURCES OF POLY- AND MONOUNSATURATED FATTY ACIDS

The main sources of polyunsaturated fatty acids are oily fish and most vegetable oils, including corn, sunflower, and safflower. The foods highest in monounsaturated fatty acids are olive and canola oils. Many nuts and seeds contain both types, some of them in a fairly balanced mixture.

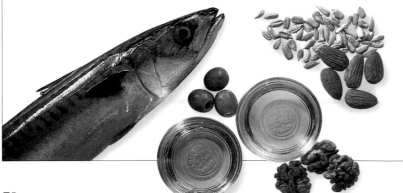

DIETARY SOURCES OF SATURATES

All animal foods are high in saturated fats. Palm and coconut oils and baked foods made with them, also have a high percentage. Saturated fats tend to be solid at room temperature.

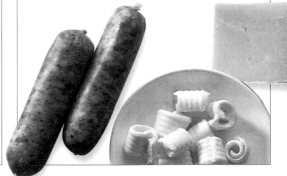

in enhancing the immune system. Cold-water fish such as salmon, mackerel, and tuna are particularly high in omega-3 fats.

Evening primrose oil is rich in the polyunsaturated fatty acid—gammalinolenic acid (GLA). In clinical studies GLA has been shown to lower cholesterol. It has also proved effective for relieving arthritis symptoms, premenstrual breast pain, and the itching of atopic eczema. Natural sources of evening primrose oil vary considerably in their GLA contents. Today a number of evening primrose oil products, most often sold in capsule form, are derived from a new cultivar that has a consistent yield of GLA.

Monounsaturated fats
Monounsaturated fats are liquid at room temperature and solid when refrigerated. They effectively lower the amount of LDLs ("bad" cholesterol) in the blood and therefore play a role in protecting against heart disease. Olive oil and some nuts are particularly high in monounsaturated fats. In Mediterranean countries such as Greece and Italy, where olive oil is used generously, the incidence of heart disease is quite low. Olive oil is believed to be one of the major factors.

Saturated fats
Saturated fats, which form a substantial proportion of the Western diet, have detrimental effects on the body. They increase the production of LDLs ("bad" cholesterol) by the liver and increase the tendency for blood to clot, which can lead to heart attack or stroke and other problems.

Animal fats are the most highly concentrated sources of saturated fats; two plant sources are palm and coconut oils. Most vegetable cooking oils, nuts, and seeds contain small amounts of saturates, and we make more in our bodies when we store fat. Saturated fats are not essential to the body, but it is hard to live without them because they are part of so many foods.

Trans fats
Trans fatty acids are formed as a result of hydrogenation, which chemically alters vegetable oils during production of margarine and shortening, changing them from liquids to solids. They also occur naturally, in small amounts, in red meat and dairy products. Studies suggest that trans fatty acids may raise LDLs and lower HDLs as much as, maybe even more than, saturated fats. In a report that came out of Harvard University, it was estimated that 30,000 deaths from heart attacks in the United States each year may be due to trans fats.

It may not be possible to avoid trans fats totally, but you can minimize your use of products that are likely to contain them. These include margarine, especially the brick type; baked goods made with shortening or margarine; and fried foods that may have been cooked in shortening.

ACHIEVING A HEALTHY BALANCE
There are many ways to cut down on both total and saturated fat and still have appealing, healthful meals and snacks.
• Substitute low-fat or nonfat dairy products and mayonnaise for their higher-fat counterparts. When you do use butter or whole-milk cheeses, do so sparingly.
• Choose lean cuts of meat with all visible fat cut away. Better still, eat fish more often, especially the cold-water types.
• Broil, microwave, steam, or bake foods rather than frying them, and when you cook with oil, choose one high in unsaturates, such as olive, sunflower, or corn oil.
• For snacks, choose fresh or dried fruit, rice cakes, air-popped popcorn with minimal or no butter, and low-fat crackers and chips.
• Use reduced-fat or nonfat salad dressings.

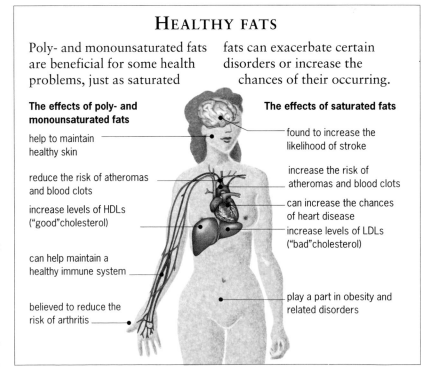

HEALTHY FATS

Poly- and monounsaturated fats are beneficial for some health problems, just as saturated fats can exacerbate certain disorders or increase the chances of their occurring.

The effects of poly- and monounsaturated fats

help to maintain healthy skin

reduce the risk of atheromas and blood clots

increase levels of HDLs ("good"cholesterol)

can help maintain a healthy immune system

believed to reduce the risk of arthritis

The effects of saturated fats

found to increase the likelihood of stroke

increase the risk of atheromas and blood clots

can increase the chances of heart disease

increase levels of LDLs ("bad"cholesterol)

play a part in obesity and related disorders

SEMI-SUPERFOODS

Certain herbs and spices, garlic, yeast, and vinegar all have healing benefits, but because of their limited nutritional content, they are not considered superfoods.

Carminatives

Flatulence, the presence of gas in the stomach or bowel, is said to be relieved by herbs called carminatives. Cardamom, dill, ginger, caraway, coriander, aniseed, fennel, nutmeg, cinnamon, and peppermint all contain volatile oils that act as carminatives.

Some of the plants and other natural products used to flavor or preserve foods also have additional benefits. Herbs—plant leaves—and spices—the bark, seeds, fruit, flower parts, or roots—have been used for thousands of years for their medicinal properties. So, too, have garlic, onions, wine, and vinegar. None of them provide much nutritional or energy value; although some do contain B vitamins and minerals such as iron, the amounts are too small to be significant. Nonetheless, they can have a potent effect on the body.

HERBS

Scientific research into the medicinal value of herbs is ongoing. While some age-old claims have been verified in the laboratory or in studies with humans, others have been discounted for lack of significanat evidence. Closer examination of some herbs has revealed possible toxic effects, and they are no longer recommended by herbalists.

A number of pharmaceutical drugs have been derived from herbs, yet it is only the drugs that have been subjected to trials, rarely the original source. Much of the evidence put forward for the healing properties of herbs is therefore anecdotal or based on the clinical experience of practitioners of herbal medicine. Countries like China have a long history of herbal medicine, while in some European countries, such as Germany and Switzerland, herbal medicines are often prescribed by orthodox medical doctors.

With or without scientific backup, millions of people champion the use of herbs and have found them to be beneficial in a variety of ways. However, many herbal remedies should be used only with the guidance of a qualified herbalist because they are powerful and can be toxic in the wrong doses or react badly with conventional medicines. On these pages only culinary herbs are included. They are used for minor complaints and for this purpose are usually taken as teas (see page 82).

Some of the herbs recommended for general digestive problems tend to have a carminative effect; that is, they release gas trapped in the intestines or stomach. Such herbs include basil and bay, which are also used to flavor soups, stews, and casseroles; chives, which have a mild onion taste and are added sometimes to soups and salads; ginger, a well-known ingredient in stir-fries, curries, and cookies; and oregano, popular in pasta sauces, casseroles, and pizzas. Also recommended for indigestion are peppermint, rosemary, and sage; these last two are often used to enhance meat, poultry, and potato dishes.

HERBAL REMEDIES FOR DIGESTIVE PROBLEMS

The painful symptoms of many digestive complaints, from indigestion to irritable bowel syndrome, can be relieved with herbal concoctions, particularly those made from essential oils.

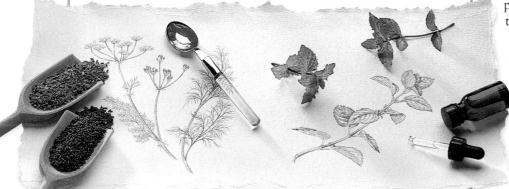

Dill and caraway A tea made with dill and caraway or fennel seeds is an aga-old remedy for relieving colic in babies or gas in adults.

Peppermint oil A tincture of peppermint oil or a tea made with peppermint leaves can help relieve indigestion.

Herbs for nondigestive problems

Oregano may ease the general symptoms of coughs and colds, while aromatic cardamom and hot chilies may relieve nasal congestion. The nervous system, too, can be affected by herbs. Basil, widely used to flavor soups, salads, and pasta dishes, is sometimes employed as an antidepressant and general tonic and may have a calming effect. Rosemary, a favorite for lamb and chicken dishes, is recommended by some herbalists for relieving headaches or promoting menstruation. It is also a natural preservative, as effective as certain synthetic antioxidants used to prevent food spoilage.

SPICES

Spices that have been found to relieve general digestive problems include turmeric, used for flavoring curries and for adding color to rice, and cayenne pepper, which can be used to add a touch of spice to any savory dish. Cayenne also stimulates gastric secretions. Cinnamon, nutmeg, and the highly aromatic cardamom are all widely used to relieve the discomfort of indigestion.

Two other digestive tonics—nutmeg, a popular flavoring for cakes and custards, and ginger, used in cakes, cookies, curries, and stir-fries—are both recommended also to relieve nausea, especially that associated with traveling and morning sickness.

The seeds of dill, caraway, and fennel, popular for flavoring fish dishes, coleslaw, bread, and pickles, are known to relieve flatulence. Cinnamon and nutmeg, used in cakes and puddings, and cumin, a flavoring for curries and casseroles, act as carminatives and digestive stimulants as well.

While many spices have the benefits named above, certain ones also have a downside and should be used with caution by some people. Chilies, for example, can cause excessive sweating and digestive problems and even precipitate diarrhea in those who are not used to them. Hot spices can also cause heartburn. If you suffer from this problem, you should avoid chilies, including cayenne. People who have peptic ulcers have always been told to avoid spices, but it now appears that ulcers are mainly caused by bacteria and that some spices may help the digestive system. Consult your doctor or a nutritionist about the pros and cons.

Spices and nondigestive problems

Both cayenne pepper and ginger are strong circulatory stimulants. Ginger also reduces the inflammation of arthritis and lowers cholesterol levels and high blood pressure. In addition, ginger can help relieve a chest cold because it has mild expectorant and cough suppressant properties and reduces fever by producing sweating. Anise is another expectorant and cough suppressant. Cinnamon is antibacterial and can be used on cuts.

Mustard seeds, favored as a spicy addition to many foods, are effective for easing muscular pains when mixed with flour and water and applied as a plaster.

GARLIC AND ONIONS

Garlic has been advocated as a remedy for various conditions for centuries. When garlic is crushed, enzymes are released that convert existing sulfur-containing compounds into a volatile, short-lived substance called allicin. Allicin has many properties, including being antibiotic, antithrombotic (preventing blood clots), and helping to reduce levels of cholesterol in the blood. Onions contain smaller amounts of allicin.

There are only a few sound studies on the biological effects of garlic, and not all the results are consistent. Large amounts of garlic need to be taken for at least six months for any effect on cholesterol levels and blood-clotting factors, after which HDLs ("good" cholesterol) levels rise, LDLs ("bad" cholesterol) levels fall and the blood tends to clot less. In Germany garlic is prescribed by doctors for lowering cholesterol levels and blood pressure. A very large European study is currently underway to assess the health effects of garlic on the heart.

Garlic is also known to have antiviral and antibiotic effects, and many people take it as a preventive or remedy for colds and flu.

Healing herbs

Below are four of the herbs and spices that have earned special recognition for their health benefits.

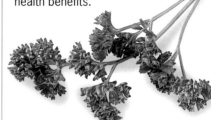

PARSLEY
This popular garnish is a proven cure for bad breath.

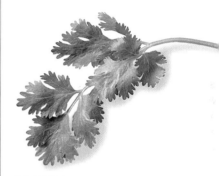

CILANTRO
This herb may be of benefit in treating amenorrhea.

SAGE
This culinary herb is effective as a gargle to ease sore throats.

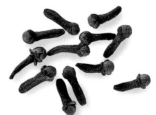

CLOVES
Oil of cloves has remarkable pain-relieving qualities that can ease toothache.

Buying and storing guide

When buying garlic, choose bulbs that have a firm head with a dry, papery sheath free of green sprouts. Garlic keeps best in a cool, dry place with good circulation. Do not refrigerate. Very fresh garlic may keep for several months.

HERBAL TEAS

Herbal teas offer a useful alternative to conventional tea and coffee because they contain very little or no tannin and no caffeine. The tannin in tea can inhibit the absorption of iron from foods, and the caffeine in both tea and coffee acts as a diuretic, leaching valuable minerals from the system, particularly potassium and calcium.

Also, caffeine stimulates the heart and nervous system, and too much of it can cause palpitations and anxiety. Replacing tea or coffee with herbal tea will ensure that your body makes the most of a meal. A wide variety of herb and fruit teas is now readily available in supermarkets. Fruit teas contain a base herb, such as hibiscus flower, and fruit flavorings. They very rarely contain the fruit itself. Herbal teas can be beneficial in a number of ways. Chamomile tea is well known for its sedative effect, as well as for relieving menstrual cramps. Try it before going to bed if you occasionally have trouble sleeping. Peppermint, fennel, and raspberry teas have long been recommended for aiding digestion and easing bloating.

Although many herbalists recommend homemade teas over store-bought ones, it is important not to use fresh herbs for teas unless you are completely sure about what you are taking and that you are using the correct part of the plant. Whenever you do use fresh herbs, make sure that you wash them thoroughly.

One safe homemade tea is ginger; infuse one or two peeled slices of fresh ginger in boiling water for 10 minutes and add a little honey to taste. Ginger is used to prevent and treat nausea and is ideal for morning sickness. It also helps relieve the chills and congestion of a cold.

ALCOHOLIC DRINKS

There is no dispute that heavy alcohol consumption is linked with increased mortality rates. Excessive drinking over time damages the heart, brain, and liver and increases the risk of many cancers, stroke, and dementia. It can also cause weight problems. Many heavy drinkers are underweight because they substitute alcohol for food; others are overweight because alcohol is high in calories, providing 7 calories per gram. On the other hand, alcohol in very moderate quantities appears to have some health benefits.

Various studies have shown that moderate alcohol consumption is associated with a lowered risk of heart disease. Regular consumption of no more than one or two drinks of alcohol per day (one for women, two for men) is linked to increased levels of the beneficial HDLs ("good" cholesterol) associated with a reduced risk of heart disease. Alcohol is also thought to reduce the stickiness of the blood, or its tendency to clot, reducing the likelihood of heart attack.

The type of alcoholic drink makes no difference, but the amount does. One drink is equal to 12 ounces of beer, 4 ounces of wine, or 1½ ounces of 80-proof liquor in a mixed drink, such as gin and tonic.

Beer

Nutritionally, beer of any sort contains calories and very little else. But it is a commonly held belief that stout is a good source of iron, an opinion that came about largely because of its dark color. However, stout contains only 0.12 milligrams of iron per 8-ounce glass, compared with beers and ales which contain 0.02 to 0.07 milligrams, so the difference is not significant.

Wine

Red wines contain flavonoids, which act as antioxidants (see page 50). Consumption of red wine may contribute to a lower incidence of heart disease in moderate wine drinkers. White wine also contains flavonoids but in smaller amounts.

HERBAL TEAS
Herbal teas are prepared by steeping fresh or dried leaves, flowers, seeds, or roots of a plant in boiling water, then straining the liquid. Usually 1 or 2 tablespoons of a dried herb are used per cup; double the amount for a fresh herb. From the top: sedative chamomile, digestion-relieving peppermint, stomach-settling ginger, and fennel to ease bloating.

> ### DID YOU KNOW?
> Too much alcohol not only damages the heart and liver but also causes problems with metabolizing glucose and numerous vitamins and minerals in the body. (Many alcoholics are malnourished for this reason.) In addition, alcohol reduces blood flow to the brain and is toxic to brain cells. Long-term overindulgence can result in memory loss, nerve damage, and even dementia.

Wine is known to be an aid to digestion because it increases production of gastrin, a digestive hormone. In addition, it stimulates the appetite, which may be useful for under-nourished people or those with a depressed appetite. A glass of wine 20 minutes before eating is advised for appetite stimulation.

A 1995 British study demonstrated the ability of both red and white wines to reduce the numbers of harmful bacteria present in contaminated water. The study also showed that neither pure alcohol nor tequila had this effect. This antimicrobial effect may explain why wine is thought to prevent traveler's diarrhea.

A glass of wine with a meal will not do any harm and may indeed do some good but should not be drunk in the belief that it is a superfood. And whatever alcohol you drink, remember that it must be spread out. Heavy drinking sessions actually damage the body.

YEAST

Yeast is a single-cell fungus that can multiply rapidly and is used to leaven bread. Although it is unusual to encounter yeast in the diet in its own right, it is a rich source of the B vitamins—thiamine (B_1), nicotinic acid, riboflavin (B_2), folate, pyridoxine (B_6), pantothenic acid, and biotin—which the body needs for the production of energy from nutrients. Yeast is low in vitamin B_{12}, but some yeast extracts are fortified with it.

The B vitamins aid the nervous and digestive systems, and some are required to maintain a healthy mouth and skin. These vitamins are also important in the production of sex hormones and red blood cells, and folic acid is essential for the prevention of neural tube defects in an unborn baby. Yeast is a reasonable source of potassium, magnesium, and zinc, all of which are important for many bodily functions, and some are also enriched with chromium, vital for the body's utilization of glucose.

Yeast is found in a variety of foods but principally in breads, pizza dough, crackers, and other baked goods. Some fermented foods also contain yeast, including cheeses, yogurt, alcoholic beverages, overripe fruit, soy sauce, vinegar, and pickled foods. One ounce of brewer's yeast, available in health food stores, contains 11 grams of protein plus 60 milligrams of vitamin C and the B vitamins listed above. Some people take brewer's yeast as a supplement.

Pathway to health

Vinegar has many uses in natural medicine and can help relieve the symptoms of a surprisingly diverse range of complaints.

To reduce foot odor, add 125 ml (½ cup) cider or white vinegar to a small tub of warm water and soak the feet for 15 minutes a day. This will also help fight fungal infections.

To soothe sunburn, add 1 cup of white vinegar to a cool bath and soak the affected area.

For vaginitis, add 3 cups of cider vinegar to warm bath water and soak for 20 minutes. This will restore normal acidity.

People who suffer from yeast allergies should use vinegar with caution because they may also be sensitive to vinegar.

VINEGAR

For more than 5,000 years people have been using vinegar to preserve food and give it an agreeably sour taste. For just as long, they have been finding other uses, from relieving headaches and sore muscles and joints to treating colds, head lice, and indigestion.

There are many types of vinegar, and all contain very few calories and no significant nutrients. However, when added to other foods, vinegar kills a wide variety of fungi and bacteria. It is this quality that has inspired many of its medicinal uses. Distilled white, the most potent vinegar, is the one most often recommended for medicinal purposes, although many people prefer cider vinegar, which is said to stimulate metabolism, aid digestion, and help the body eliminate toxins. Some people who suffer with arthritis have found that a tonic of cider vinegar and honey helps relieve pain.

Three proven vinegar remedies are: relief of sunburn and insect bites, treatment of athlete's foot, and prevention of swimmer's ear, a painful infection of the inner ear. To prevent a waterlogged ear from becoming infected, doctors advise mixing isopropyl alcohol with an equal amount of white vinegar and adding the mixture to the ear with a dropper. (Note: This should not be done if the eardrum has burst.)

Yeast allergy

Some people are allergic to yeast, and this can cause a rash and possibly eczema. Yeast extract contains chemicals called vasoactive amines, which may dilate blood vessels. Other foods rich in vasoactive amines are chocolate, cheese, red wine, and citrus fruits. These foods can cause facial flushing and headaches and may be a major trigger for migraines in certain people. Vasoactive amines can also constrict blood vessels in some cases and affect the nervous system. Because many foods contain yeast, always check food labels if you are allergic to it.

VINEGAR HAIR WASH
To treat dandruff, add 1 tablespoon of cider vinegar to a pint of warm water and use as a rinse after shampooing.

HEALTH CLAIMS AND FOOD FACTS

Where do you turn when you want a quick burst of energy or a genuine blood-pressure reducer? Knowing what certain foods can do will help you plan the best possible diet.

There are various foods that you simply do not need, including sugar with its empty calories, and algae with their widely claimed super powers. And there are foods that may cause harm when eaten in excess or by pregnant women.

SUGARS

Sugars are simple carbohydrates that taste sweet and provide quick energy bursts but do not supply any other nutrients. There are many types of sweeteners, including sucrose (table sugar), fructose (in honey and fruits), glucose (in honey, fruits, and vegetables), and lactose (in milk). Refined sugars, which provide only empty calories, should be kept to a minimum in the diet; in fact, many people should cut their intake of refined sugar by 50 percent. The sugars in fruits and sweet vegetables like beets can be consumed on a regular basis because they are bound up with essential vitamins, minerals, and fiber.

Each gram of sugar provides four calories of energy and no other nutrients. Sugar is added to many processed foods and may be described on the ingredients list as sucrose, glucose, dextrose, maltose, or fructose. Indeed, half the sugar in the average diet is added to foods by food manufacturers. The other half comes from what is added in the home kitchen or at the table.

Sometimes a quick burst of energy from sugar is just what you need, but for sustained energy you should turn to the complex carbohydrates in starchy foods like bread. Too often sugary foods replace more nutritious ones in the diet and result in ill health and overweight. Foods that contain large amounts of refined sugar are also the main cause of tooth decay because bacteria in the plaque on teeth turn the sugar into acid, which in turn attacks tooth enamel.

Sugar does have some positive uses. It can be incorporated in a wound dressing (see sidebar, opposite page) or used as a preservative in jams and syrups, and when added to tart fruits, it makes them more palatable. It also provides pleasure, lifting the mood when nothing else seems capable of doing so.

Honey

It is a common belief that honey has some nutritive value because it is eaten in its natural state. In fact, it has only traces of nutrients and, volume for volume, is higher in calories than white sugar. However, because it is sweeter, a smaller amount is needed to achieve the same sweetness as with sugar (1 part honey to 1¼ parts sugar). But sugar does not have honey's complex flavors. Honey can be used in baking as an alternative to sugar. Cakes and pastries that include

SWEET STUFF
Simple sugars come in many guises, so much so that some people believe certain types to be healthier than others. In fact, the honey, corn syrup, brown sugar, and turbinado crystals shown here are no better for health than the white sugar cubes.

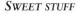

The better choice

Many foods have had health benefits attributed to them over the centuries. Some of the claims have stood up to rigorous scientific testing in recent years but many have not. At worst, these foods simply do not have the beneficial effects claimed for them. At best, they have some merit but are less useful than other foods in promoting good health. A few of the myths are unveiled below.

Ginseng may boost the immune system and improve stamina and concentration, but it may also lead to insomnia. It is prefereable to rely on foods rich in B vitamins and potassium, such as bananas, meat, and milk.

Sugars may supply quick energy in the short term, but the more slowly absorbed complex carbohydrates, such as those in bread and other cereal foods and starchy vegetables, give a longer-lasting energy boost.

Shiitake mushrooms can help lower blood cholesterol levels, but portions are generally too small to have a significant impact. It's better to stick to a low-fat and low-cholesterol diet that includes a regular intake of legumes like peas.

honey tend to remain moister for a longer period of time because of honey's capacity to retain water.

Although honey has an age-old reputation for its healing qualities, many of the claims have not been medically proved. Honey's most popular medicinal uses are for sore throats and coughs. In fact, it is a common ingredient in cough lozenges, and when added to hot water with a little lemon juice, is very soothing for a sore throat. Like table sugar, it also has antiseptic properties and helps wounds to heal.

Various claims for royal jelly (used to feed the queen bee) as a cure-all and revitalizer are not proven. In fact, it may provoke asthmatic attacks in some people.

Molasses and raw sugar
Molasses is a thick, sweet, strong-flavored substance that is extracted during the early stages of sugar refining. One tablespoon of molasses contains 1 milligram of iron (one tenth of the RDA for men), 300 milligrams of potassium, and 42 milligrams of calcium, plus traces of other minerals. Brown sugar is made by coating white sugar with molasses, but the amount is too small to be of nutritional value.

What some people call raw sugar is actually turbinado, raw sugar that has been purified. (Raw sugar is not sold in the United States because it is contaminated with soil, plant refuse, and insect droppings.)

Sugar substitutes
There are two groups of sugar substitutes. The first, consisting of sugar alcohols, includes names that may be familiar from food labels, such as mannitol, xylitol, and maltilol. The second includes the artificial sweeteners aspartame, saccharin, and acesulfame-K.

The sugar alcohols contain as many calories as sucrose and are therefore not beneficial if you are trying to substitute sugar in order to lose weight. They do, however, have one important advantage over sugar: they can reduce tooth decay; for this reason, many dentists recommend chewing sugar-free gum containing sorbitol after meals.

Artificial sweeteners have virtually no calories and are far sweeter than sugar. Various claims have been made that link saccharin with cancer and aspartame with headaches and vision problems, but there is no conclusive evidence to date. Some studies also indicate that these supersweet substances may actually increase a craving for

Wound dressings
Sugar is an effective wound healer. Certain wounds, such as varicose ulcers and severe burns, are normally very slow to heal, and the problem is compounded by damage caused when old dressings are removed. A paste made from sugar, when applied to wounds under a waterproof dressing, accelerates healing because of its ability to draw out moisture and inhibit the growth of bacteria. These simple but very effective dressings are widely used today by doctors.

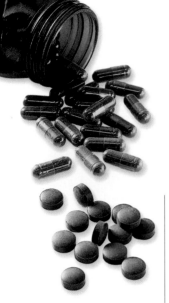

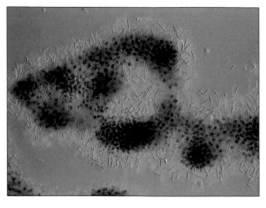

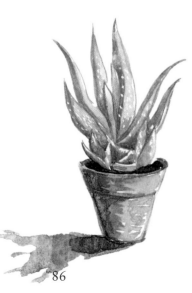

CURE-ALL ALGAE?
The picture above right is a light micrograph, magnified 200 times, of chlorella, a green alga that inhabits ponds and lakes. This and another alga, spirulina, are available in tablet form and have an effect similar to that of a multivitamin. However, great health and cure-all claims made for them have proved unfounded.

ALOE VERA
Applied to the skin, aloe vera has healing properties. The dried sap of the leaf is also used as a laxative by some people.

sweets. Used in moderation, however, they seem to be effective sugar substitutes.

EXOTIC FOODS

There are foods not widely included in Western diets that have had great health claims made about them. Although some of these remain scientifically unproven, many people believe in them, and a few are still being studied.

Spirulina and chlorella

Two algae, spirulina and chlorella, are gathered from freshwater lakes in the tropics or cultivated commercially in several places, including Thailand, Japan, Mexico, and southern California. They are often taken as supplements in powder and tablet forms.

It has been claimed that ginseng can restore vitality and act as a general stimulant because it contains complex chemical substances known as ginsenosides. In the Far East ginseng has been used as a tea for thousands of years to extend youthful vigor

They contain the B-complex vitamins and beta carotene. Spirulina is also claimed to be a good source of gamma linolenic acid (GLA), which is an essential fatty acid. Various health claims have been made for spirulina and chlorella, including that they act as energy boosters, help control weight, detoxify the body, and boost the immune system. None of these benefits has been proved. Both supplements are expensive, and though they provide some vitamins, they are not a magic cure.

Ginseng

Ginseng preparations are made from the dried root of the ginseng plant. The best-known and most effective species are *Panax ginseng,* which grows in China, the central Himalayas, Japan, and Korea, and *Panax quinquefolius,* its North American cousin.

and improve libido. There is some scientific evidence to show that ginseng can improve stamina, concentration, and appetite, while other research indicates that the herb can boost immunity. However, if taken in excess, it can lead to insomnia or other nervous disturbances. Ginseng does have some effects that mimic those of the female sex hormone estrogen, so some women use it during menopause. Ginseng is usually taken in tablet form in the West and can be found in health food stores and pharmacies.

Shiitake mushrooms

Often used in Japanese and Chinese cooking, shiitake mushrooms have a rich flavor. Asian herbalists advocate eating shiitakes for a healthy and long life. Claims have also been made that shiitakes can lower blood cholesterol levels and boost the immune system when eaten in large enough amounts. Like all mushrooms, shiitakes are good sources of potassium and trace elements. They are also low in fat and calories unless, of course, they are fried.

In practice, however, mushrooms tend to be eaten in small amounts and therefore do not make a significant contribution to diet except in providing variety.

In the dried form, which is the way they are most often sold, shiitake mushrooms need to be soaked before use. Either soak them in cold water for an hour or soften them in very hot water for 25 to 30 minutes. Once soft they should be squeezed dry and the hard stems discarded. The soaking liquid can be strained and added to the dish in which the mushrooms are being used.

Aloe vera

A distinctive plant with pointed, fleshy leaves (see far left), aloe vera is a member of the *Aloe* genus, many members of which are cultivated as a source of laxatives. Aloe vera is not grown here for this purpose, but it is a common ingredient in soothing skin lotions and other cosmetic products.

You can use fresh aloe vera directly on sunburn, rashes, cuts, and scrapes; break open a leaf and squeeze the gel onto the affected area. Some herbalists advocate taking aloe vera juice or tablets as a tonic, slimming aid, or arthritis treatment, but there is no scientific evidence for such claims. In fact, when taken orally, aloe vera can interfere with the body's absorption of iron and other minerals because of its tannin content.

Menu Planning

Because no single food provides all the nutrients your body needs, you should eat a variety of foods for optimum health. The suggestions below may serve as starting points; you can tailor them to suit your own tastes and needs.

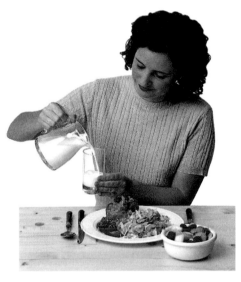

One way to make sure that your diet balances well is to plan meals for several days at a time. If you miss out on some basic nutrients one day, you can make up the difference on another day. Also, you can see if you are getting enough variety overall. It is not necessary to group your foods into three meals; spread them over four to six if it's more convenient.

The goal for each day should be
• at least 5 servings of bread, cereal, rice, and other starchy foods
• 3 to 5 servings of vegetables
• 2 to 4 servings of fruit
• 1 to 2 servings of meat, poultry, fish, eggs, or high-protein alternatives such as dried legumes and nuts
• 2 to 3 servings of dairy products or calcium-fortified foods

UNENDING CHOICES
Keep adding new foods to your menus and make sure you have a balance of all food groups every day.

HEALTHY MEALS THROUGHOUT THE DAY

Breakfasts

If you often skip breakfast because you have no time in the morning, prepare it before you go to bed at night. Also, stock up on foods you can take to work or school when there is no time for breakfast.

High-fiber breakfast cereals, such as oatmeal or bran flakes, served with nonfat or low-fat milk provide a great start to the day. Add dried or fresh fruit for additional nutrients and flavor. If you don't like milk on cereal, try fruit juice instead.

To start your day with a good supply of protein, cook eggs any way you like them and serve with whole-grain bread; or make grilled cheese and tomatoes on a sprouted wheat bagel; or toast country bread and spread it with peanut butter.

For a fruity breakfast, try a spiced dried-fruit compote or a bowl of exotic fresh fruits with low-fat yogurt to boost your calcium intake.

You don't have to limit yourself to typical breakfast foods. Eating leftovers from dinner can be a great way to start the day.

Lunches and snacks

If you favor sandwiches for lunch, make them work in your nutritional favor. Use mostly whole-grain breads and avoid high-fat luncheon meats for fillings, using instead fish, chicken breast, low-fat cheese, or beans plus leafy greens and other vegetables. If you are toting lunch to work or school, pack the vegetables separately and add them to the sandwich at the last minute.

Some new twists on old standbys for sandwich fillings are tuna with plain nonfat yogurt, chopped cucumber or red onion, and dill; peanut butter with shredded carrot, chopped celery, sliced apple, chopped dried fruit, or raisins.

For a satisfying lunchtime meal, try a baked potato topped with chili con carne, cheese and broccoli, baked beans, or cottage cheese.

A bowl of vegetable soup with a whole-grain bread or roll could not be better for lunch.

For a super snack, try air-popped popcorn with a light coating of butter-flavored nonstick cooking spray.

Main courses

As you think about weekly menus, you can make life easier for yourself by planning main-course dishes that will do double duty at other meals. For example, when you prepare meat or vegetables for dinner, cook twice as much as you need and use the leftovers to add to salad, soup, a sandwich, or a pasta dish the next day.

Try to include seafood on the daily menu at least twice a week.

Make a starchy food such as rice, pasta, or potatoes the basis of most main courses, using meat, fish, or legumes as accompaniments.

DESSERTS
Fruit-based desserts, such as crumbles, fruited yogurt or frozen yogurt, sorbet, or fresh fruit topped with low-fat custard can all be part of a healthful diet.

Excellent apples

The ancient Greeks believed that apples cured all ailments. Apples do have health benefits—they are low in calories and high in soluble fiber, which helps control blood cholesterol levels and prevent constipation. Also, chewing an apple stimulates saliva flow, which lowers levels of decay-causing bacteria. But apples will not, as claimed by *American Medicine* in 1927, help with nervous and skin diseases, rheumatism, or "autointoxication."

If you decide to take aloe vera internally, it is important to remember that, like other aloe species, it contains laxative compounds, which can disturb the absorption of fluids, electrolytes, and other nutrients. If you are at all concerned, check with your doctor or a qualified herbalist.

OLD FAVORITES

Huge numbers of health claims have been made about foods that are favorites in the Western diet. However, a certain amount of fiction or exaggeration is mixed with the facts, and we still have much to learn.

Beans

Claims have been made that beans help combat depression. There is no evidence of their having a direct impact on this condition, but beans—in fact, all legumes—are good sources of vitamin B_6, folate, and selenium, all of which are important to proper nerve function, particularly creation of mood-lifting neurotransmitters. In two separate studies, depressed patients given folate supplements showed marked improvement, and a group of people deficient in selenium improved in mood with selenium supplements.

Cherries

Cherries were once claimed to cure kidney stones, epilepsy, and gallbladder problems, and to relieve gout. There is no proof to back up the first three claims, but some people with gout have had good results from drinking two glasses a day of cherry juice.

Chili peppers

Eclectic physicians of the 19th century recommended chili peppers to relieve constipation, toothache, nausea, and diarrhea, and to stimulate the circulatory and digestive systems. They also advised its use externally to relieve arthritis and muscle soreness. These last two are now proven remedies. A gargle made with chilies will ease a sore throat.

Chocolate

Many people eat chocolate to give themselves a mental lift, which possibly results from the caffeine it contains. However, the amount of caffeine in most chocolate is too small to have a significant effect. Chocolate is also rich in phenylethylamine, a compound that has effects similar to those of amphetamine. Recent research indicates that chocolate has certain health benefits when eaten in moderate amounts.

Spinach

Popeye was wrong! Spinach is highly nutritious but is not a miracle food that will increase one's strength. It is a good source of iron, however. A 4-ounce serving contains 4 mg of iron—nearly half of the recommended daily intake for men.

THE TRUTH ABOUT SUPERFOODS

A treasure trove of superfoods would be a delight to all, but unfortunately, many claims about certain foods seem to be based more on fantasy than fact.

Including superfoods regularly in your diet will certainly do you good. However, the best approach to achieving optimal health is to eat a wide variety of foods.

BENEFITS . . .

Dried fruits provide iron and other minerals.

Chili peppers may help prevent blood clots; can help relieve nasal congestion.

Apples contain ample soluble fiber to lower blood cholesterol; their low calories aid in weight loss.

Spinach can help prevent cancer with its antioxidants and anemia with its iron.

Beans can help lower blood cholesterol, regulate insulin, and boost fiber levels.

LIMITATIONS . . .

Stickiness can cause tooth decay.

They are not useful as a general tonic; can irritate eyes.

They are relatively low in nutrients.

The oxalic acid in spinach hinders absorption of its minerals.

Beans won't beat depression but can improve mood.

CHAPTER 5

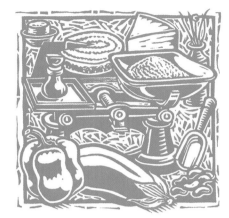

MANAGING ILLNESS WITH FOOD

*Just as food can affect your health
if you have too few nutrients or the wrong
balance of them, it can help along the natural
process of healing when you become ill. Certain
foods contain nutrients that are necessary
for healing, while others, when restricted
or eliminated from your diet, may speed
recovery. Some foods can also be useful
when applied externally as poultices.*

FOOD AND HEALING

Food has been used for healing throughout history. Scientific explanations for many of their healing properties are leading today to the increasing use of food for relieving illness.

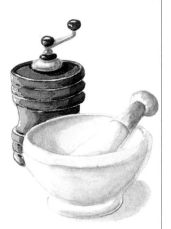

SPICE REMEDIES
In Chinese medicine spices like ginger and pepper may be used to relieve chronic "cold" disorders such as poor digestion.

Two thousand years ago Hippocrates, father of Western medicine, wrote: "Let food be your medicine and medicine be your food." Indeed, long before Hippocrates' time and ever since, food has played a vital role in health care.

In both Indian and Chinese traditional medicine, foods are used for their healing properties. Chinese and Tibetan medical practitioners recommend foods to correct imbalances in the body. Their system of "hot" and "cold" foods is based on the yin and yang principles—yin equals cold; yang equals hot. Foods are categorized according to a variety of factors, such as the climate they grow in, the speed of growth, and a host of other conditions. Once the quality of a food is established, it can be used, according to these principles, to correct the body's imbalances. For example, "cold" foods such as fruits and leafy vegetables are recommended to disperse "hot" conditions like bronchitis and high blood pressure. In China today there are restaurants that offer customers an expert health assessment according to traditional medical principles and then select a menu for them.

In the Western world the use of diet for healing has for many years been the specialty of naturopathic physicians. Naturopathy is based on the principle that the human body, given the right conditions, will cure itself of illness; naturopaths focus on diet, exercise, and elimination of accumulated waste products to heal disorders. Pioneers of natural healing, such as F. E. Bilz in Germany in the late 19th century, Max Bircher-Benner in Switzerland in the early 20th century, and Stanley Lief in the United Kingdom in 1928, all established residential clinics where fasting, diet therapies, and physical treatments were used to treat a number of conditions.

PLANTS THAT HEAL FROM WITHOUT

For centuries certain food plants have been used externally for healing. They have been mashed or ground to make ointments and salves for applying topically to wounds or infections, or steeped to make poultices. Many such remedies are still used today, although more often in pursuit of beauty rather than healing.

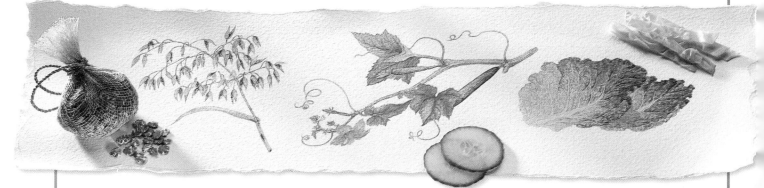

Oats can bring relief from the itching and irritation of eczema. Tie a bag of oatmeal to a bathtub faucet so that the water runs through it. Soak yourself in the tub for at least 10 minutes.

Cucumber is a favorite in beauty treatments; two slices of cucumber placed over the eyes for 15 minutes will soothe and refresh them.

Cabbage is helpful in reducing swellings, especially those that occur after injuries to joints. For best effect, apply poultices made of crushed or shredded cabbage leaves and juice.

With the development of antibiotics and painkillers in the 1950s, earlier forms of treatment were neglected, but modern research in nutritional biochemistry is validating many recommendations of the early naturopaths. For example, it is now known that vegetables of the cruciferous, or brassica, family (cabbage, cauliflower, broccoli, kale), which traditionally have been part of the raw-diet regimen recommended by naturopaths, are rich in compounds related to vitamin C that are known to help protect against inflammatory changes in the joints.

The rest of this chapter gives specific examples of how you can enhance the healing process for specific ailments by adjusting your diet. This is usually easy to do, and though many ailments can be treated or improved by changes in eating habits, it is essential that you seek a proper diagnosis.

PROFESSIONAL GUIDANCE

The recommendations in this chapter are appropriate for most people to follow, but it may be advisable to seek professional guidance for a diet tailored to your individual needs. Your body type, for example, can affect the ailments to which you may be prone, and your genes determine the various aspects of your biochemistry that make your nutritional needs unique.

When seeking professional advice, consult qualified practitioners who have the clinical skills to make a medical and nutritional assessment of your needs. Some doctors use food and nutrition to help in the management of ailments; they diagnose a patient's needs, using careful clinical examination. Practitioners may also analyze blood, urine, or sweat to determine any imbalances that can have an impact on the ability to recover from ill health.

Orthodox doctors who treat illness with changes in diet often focus on problems associated with intolerance to foods as well as environmental factors, such as exposure to chemicals and other irritants. Other health therapists, including naturopaths, homeopaths, medical herbalists, osteopaths, and chiropractors, give dietary guidance in conjunction with their main therapies. Also, dietitians and many nutritionists have special training in food chemistry and menu planning and can give you guidance about eating healthfully, as well as providing diet plans for specific illnesses.

Some doctors and health therapists recommend nutritional supplements when a situation calls for them. Additional vitamins and minerals can be beneficial when an ailment creates a greater need for them. However, a proper clinical assessment should always be done first.

Without professional advice, only a balanced vitamin and mineral supplement should be taken on a regular basis, and then only when combined with food, because the body requires a combination of nutrients to work efficiently. Taking an excess of a particular nutrient can deplete another one.

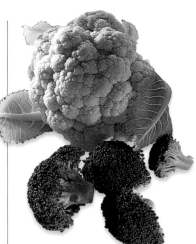

CARING CRUCIFERS
Cauliflower and broccoli, now known to be highly beneficial in the battle against cancer, have long been recommended to relieve inflammation in muscles and joints.

THE INTERACTION BETWEEN FOODS AND MEDICINE

Some medicines affect absorption of nutrients from food, possibly causing deficiencies, while some foods and vitamin supplements prevent absorption of particular medicines. Certain medicines should be taken with foods; others should not.

DRUG	TAKEN FOR	PROBLEM	ACTION
Antacids	Indigestion	May deplete phosphorus.	Eat meat, eggs, and fish.
Laxatives (used to excess)	Constipation	May deplete potassium and other nutrients.	Eat whole-grain foods, fruits, and vegetables.
Antibiotics	Illnesses and infections	May deplete friendly bacteria in the bowel.	Eat yogurt with live cultures.
Diuretics	Water retention and kidney problems	May deplete potassium and magnesium.	Eat fruits, whole grains, legumes, and vegetables.
Anticoagulants	Prevention of strokes or blood clots	Vitamin E may make their effect stronger.	Avoid taking vitamin E supplements.

Nutritional Therapy

A number of doctors and dietitians are teaming up today to help people cope with a range of disorders, from allergies to cancer to chronic headaches and sinusitis, by examining and adjusting their diets.

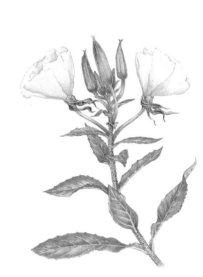

EVENING PRIMROSE OIL AND PMS
Evening primrose oil is a rich natural source of gamma linolenic acid (GLA), which is useful for relieving the pain of premenstrual breast tenderness. The oil is available in capsules from pharmacies and health food stores.

Scientific research is identifying more and more links between nutrition and disease. While many doctors and other health professionals maintain that much of this research is too inconclusive to be a basis for sound nutritional advice, others are working with patients to find nutritional routes to good health. The results have been mixed, some approaches are highly controversial, and many theories have yet to be proved with unbiased research. Yet anecdotal evidence suggests that many possibilities for preventing and/or curing disease with diet are still untapped.

What is nutritional therapy?
In some countries, the United Kingdom, for example, there is a category of health care known as nutritional therapy. While no such practice exists in the U.S., some doctors, dietitians, and nurses who have training in nutrition are helping patients with special needs to find a nutritional route to health. A number of these specialists work in teams.

Depending on their training and beliefs, some practitioners hold the view that nutritional deficiencies or toxic substances in food are causes of common illnesseses. Others advise on special dietary approaches to coping with cancer.

How do you find a nutritional therapist?
You can call a local hospital for the names of qualified practitioners. Be as specific as you can about your particular needs when you inquire.

What qualifications should a practitioner have?
Backgrounds vary. At the very least any person who is giving nutritional advice should have an undergraduate degree in food and nutritional studies and some graduate work in a nutrition specialty. A registered dietitian (R.D.) will have also done an internship in dietetics and be a member of the American Dietetics Association.

A naturopathic doctor (N.D.) will have graduated from one of two graduate schools in the United States that require four years of study and clinical experience.

Origins

Modern nutritional therapy emerged in the latter half of the 20th century as a combination of nutritional medicine, naturopathy, and clinical ecology. The first of these three, nutritional medicine, arose from research carried out after the discovery of vitamins and their ability to cure diseases like pellagra, which were not previously known to be deficiency disorders. Naturopathy, a philosophy born at the end of the 19th century, treats disease with cleansing diets, herbal remedies, and other natural methods. The clinical ecology movement began in the 1940s with American Dr. Theron G. Randolph and his interest in patients who were suffering from allergies.

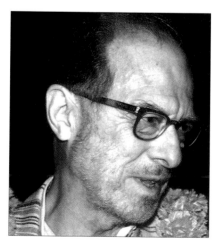

THERON G. RANDOLPH, M.D.
The discovery that at least 30 percent of his patients were suffering from allergies drew him to clinical ecology.

What will a consultation be like?
Treatment by nutritional therapy takes time and several approaches may be tried before finding the most effective one. Consultation will probably include questions about your diet, lifestyle, and habits, a physical examination of skin, tongue, nails, and hair, and additional laboratory tests, depending on the problem.

How do nutritional therapists diagnose deficiencies?
The symptoms themselves usually suggest the groups of nutrients that may be lacking. Blood and other tests can also identify a deficiency but may not reveal how severe the deficiency is. The level of certain nutrients in the blood is maintained by organs that donate their reserves. By the time a deficiency shows up in blood tests, it can be quite advanced, and side effects may already be obvious. A nutritional therapist will try to recognize the problem and offer help before this point is reached.

Surely if you eat a balanced diet you can't have deficiencies?
A great deal happens to food between the time you ingest it and the point when nutrients are finally assimilated into your body's tissues and cells. For instance, insufficient hydrochloric acid in your stomach can impair the process of digestion, or an imbalance of intestinal bacteria may hinder absorption of certain nutrients. Nutritional therapists use diets and supplements to create better conditions for digestion and absorption, helping the body to function more efficiently and heal itself.

TOXIC OVERLOAD
Many specialists in diet therapy believe that toxins come not just from pollutants that surround us but also from the use of medications, alcohol, and caffeine, from dysbiosis (a poor balance of bacteria) in the intestines, food additives, and even from food itself. The toxicity can build up and cause damage if your digestive system is not very efficient at neutralizing and eliminating these substances. A naturopath may use a variety of diets, herbs, and nutritional approaches to aid these processes and expel toxins.

WHAT YOU CAN DO
Chronic disorders, such as migraine, irritable bowel syndrome, and sinusitis can be caused or made worse by a food allergy or intolerance. Many nutritional specialists work closely with people who suffer such conditions to identify problem foods and improve resistance to them.

If you suffer from chronic ailments, try experimentally cutting out the likeliest offenders—first wheat and then dairy products—for a week each to see if your condition improves. Remember that wheat is found in bread, crackers, cakes, biscuits, puddings, sauces, and other things made from flour. Dairy products include not just milk but its derivatives such as whey and caseine. You must read product labels carefully because even tiny amounts can cause symptoms in people.

If you think you have identified a particular food as a cause of your illness, you will find it helpful to seek professional advice on menu planning. Always consult a doctor if any illness is persistent or worsens.

DETAILED EXAMINATION
Because foods can affect every aspect of the body, a doctor or naturopath who is looking for links between food and a disorder may examine you very closely, paying attention to every symptom, from fingernail condition to overall energy levels.

FATIGUE AND HEADACHES

Fatigue and headaches are suffered by many people from time to time. Usually they resolve themselves, but if they persist or become severe, then the causes need to be investigated.

Foods to avoid

Anemic people should avoid too much unprocessed bran and unleavened bread because these have a high phytic acid content that binds iron and prevents efficient absorption. Yeast used in baking breaks down phytic acid in wheat flour and releases the iron. Tannin in tea also blocks the absorption of iron.

While fatigue may be a symptom of a nutritional deficiency like anemia, there can also be other causes, such as muscular tension, postviral fatigue, or thyroid problems, and a professional diagnosis is necessary. Nevertheless, dietary management can support any medical treatment you may require.

ANEMIA

Persistent tiredness is one of the main symptoms of anemia—a deficiency of red blood cells or their oxygen-carrying compound, hemoglobin. Although there are many types of anemia and a number of causes, lack of iron in the body is the most common cause. It is essential that suspected anemia be diagnosed by a doctor so that appropriate treatment can be determined.

In addition to any supplement prescribed by your doctor (it is no longer recommended to take iron supplements except on medical advice), a diet rich in iron and other nutrients that improve the uptake of iron will speed recovery. Lean meat and green leafy vegetables (especially spinach and beet greens) are the best iron sources. Red blood cells require not just iron for healthy func-

ANEMIA AND FATIGUE

When they are formed, red blood cells are full of a protein called hemoglobin, each unit of which holds one iron ion (the part of the cell that carries oxygen).

Lack of iron reduces the amount of hemoglobin, which then diminishes the cells' capacity for oxygen. Anemic cells starve muscles of oxygen, causing tiredness

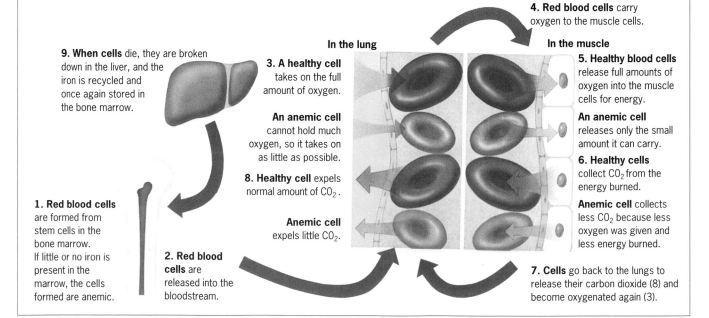

9. When cells die, they are broken down in the liver, and the iron is recycled and once again stored in the bone marrow.

1. Red blood cells are formed from stem cells in the bone marrow. If little or no iron is present in the marrow, the cells formed are anemic.

2. Red blood cells are released into the bloodstream.

In the lung

3. A healthy cell takes on the full amount of oxygen.

An anemic cell cannot hold much oxygen, so it takes on as little as possible.

8. Healthy cell expels normal amount of CO_2.

Anemic cell expels little CO_2.

4. Red blood cells carry oxygen to the muscle cells.

In the muscle

5. Healthy blood cells release full amounts of oxygen into the muscle cells for energy.

An anemic cell releases only the small amount it can carry.

6. Healthy cells collect CO_2 from the energy burned.

Anemic cell collects less CO_2 because less oxygen was given and less energy burned.

7. Cells go back to the lungs to release their carbon dioxide (8) and become oxygenated again (3).

tion but also protein (found in animal products, beans, and other legumes), folic acid (in green leafy vegetables), B vitamins (in whole grains and animal products), and vitamin C (in citrus fruits and peppers).

Iron-deficient anemia is more common in women who have heavy or prolonged menstrual periods and in the elderly, whose digestive systems absorb nutrients less efficiently. The absorption of iron is aided by vitamin C (see page 19). Poor digestion may be improved by apple cider vinegar because its acidity stimulates secretion of digestive enzymes. (Mix a teaspoon of apple cider vinegar in a glass of warm water, add a little honey to taste, and drink before every meal.)

Vegetarians and vitamin B$_{12}$

People who convert to vegetarian diets should be concerned about their levels of vitamin B$_{12}$. This vitamin is found primarily in meat, fish, and some dairy foods, but most plants do not contain any. Vitamin B$_{12}$ is necessary for energy production and healthy development of the nervous system and red blood cells. A deficiency can cause a serious disorder called pernicious anemia.

The body stores vitamin B$_{12}$ for three to five years, so for vegetarians who eat few animal proteins, or vegans who eat none at all, the signs of deficiency, such as fatigue, poor concentration, and weakness, may become evident only after some years.

B$_{12}$ deficiency can be prevented by a sufficiently varied diet that includes dairy foods and eggs and, particularly for vegans, such fermented soy products as tofu, miso, and tempeh. Vegans can also drink soy milk enriched with B$_{12}$.

CHRONIC FATIGUE SYNDROME (POSTVIRAL FATIGUE)

Fatigue that cannot be attributed to diseases of the blood, such as anemia, or to thyroid problems or other distinct disorders is sometimes labeled postviral fatigue syndrome because the onset often follows a viral illness. In the United States it was

WARM CHICKEN LIVER SALAD

Liver is an excellent source of iron (a 2-ounce serving of chicken livers contains almost 5 mg) and is particularly good for people who are trying to rebuild their iron stores after being diagnosed with anemia.

1 head curly endive (chicory)
½ bunch watercress
100 g/4 oz mushrooms, wiped and sliced
50 g/2 oz raisins
225 g/8 oz chicken livers
2 tbsp sunflower oil
1 shallot, peeled and finely sliced
2 tbsp red wine vinegar
freshly ground black pepper and salt to taste

■ Wash the curly endive and watercress, tear into small pieces, and mix with the mushrooms and raisins. Arrange on four plates.
■ In a medium skillet, heat the oil and cook the shallot over low heat until softened.
■ Wash, trim, and dry the chicken livers on paper towels, then halve them. Add the livers to the pan with the shallots and cook for 5 minutes, stirring all the time, until browned.
■ Remove from the pan with a slotted spoon and divide among the plates of salad.
■ Add the vinegar, pepper, and salt to the pan, stirring to scrape up any browned bits. Bring the mixture to a boil and then drizzle some over each salad. Serve immediately.
Serves 4

named after the most common of these, the Epstein-Barr virus, which causes glandular fever. In the United Kingdom the syndrome became known as myalgic encephalomyelitis (ME). All these terms have now been replaced by the name chronic fatigue syndrome (CFS).

Symptoms include a debilitating tiredness, often worse after exercise, muscular aches, headaches, recurring sore throats, painful large glands in the neck, and poor concentration. The desire to do things but the physical inability to be active distinguishes CFS from depression, with which CFS sufferers are sometimes mistakenly diagnosed. If you have CFS, some of the dietary measures described below may aid your recovery.

It is possible that some sufferers of CFS have low blood sugar or functional hypoglycemia (see page 96). They may also have intestinal candidiasis, an overgrowth of a certain yeast in the gut, which worsens the fatigue and hinders recovery .

Lactic fermented foods, such as yogurt with live cultures and sauerkraut, are thought to promote the growth of lactic acid bacteria in the gut, which help protect

MUESLI

A hearty muesli—full of wheat, oats, rye, nuts, seeds, and dried fruits—topped with a selection of seasonal fresh fruits supplies vitamins and minerals necessary for health, as well as complex carbohydrates for sustained energy.

225 g/8 oz rolled oats
175 g/6 oz wheat flakes
175 g/6 oz rye flakes
175 g/6 oz barley flakes
100 g/4 oz sunflower
   seeds
100 g/4 oz hazelnuts,
   chopped
100 g/4 oz dried dates,
   chopped
100 g/4 oz dried
   apricots, chopped
100 g/4 oz dried prunes,
   pitted and chopped
100 g/4 oz raisins

■ Mix all the ingredients together and store in an airtight container. Serve with fresh fruits and plain low-fat yogurt, low-fat or nonfat milk, or fruit juice.
Makes 1.5 kg/3 lb 2 oz, about 40 servings

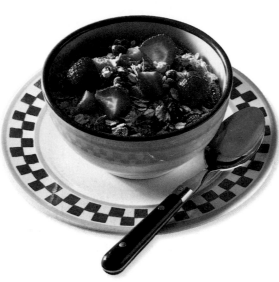

INSULIN
The hexagonal shapes (below) are molecules of the hormone insulin. Produced in the pancreas, this hormone regulates the level of sugar in the blood.

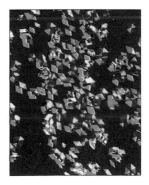

against yeast overgrowth. If you suspect that you have low blood sugar or intestinal candidiasis, you should consult a doctor who practices nutritional medicine or a naturopath and arrange for the necessary laboratory tests that can identify these problems.

A deficiency of magnesium has been associated with CFS. Increasing your intake of magnesium-rich foods, such as green leafy vegetables, millet and other whole grains, legumes, and brown rice, will help replenish it. Increasing foods that are rich in antioxidants, such as vitamins E and C and beta carotene will also be helpful. These include wheat germ, green leafy vegetables, nuts, and seeds (for E); fruits, peppers, potatoes, and broccoli (for C), and orange fruits and vegetables (for beta carotene).

LOW BLOOD SUGAR

Low blood sugar, or functional hypoglycemia, is an imbalance in the body's energy-producing processes. It is a common cause of fatigue and headaches when blood sugar levels drop sharply, and deprives the brain of its essential fuel.

Blood sugar levels normally drop after extra physical or emotional demands and after long periods of time without eating. A consistently low level of blood sugar, however, is believed to be caused by oversensitivity of the pancreas, which secretes the hormone insulin to convert sugar to energy. This process can be overstimulated by a diet that is high in alcohol, refined sugar, and stimulants like caffeine.

Within two or three hours of eating a large amount of refined sugar or other concentrated sucrose, such as that in honey, the blood-sugar level will plunge because of the excessive insulin out put by the overworked pancreas. This means that chocolate and other sweets will improve your energy in the short term, but they can actually make you feel more tired later on. Because they are such concentrated forms of sugar, these foods are absorbed rapidly into the bloodstream and induce the release of an excessive amount of the sugar-utilizing hormone insulin. This can cause blood sugar levels to swing from high to low and back and rapidly lead to an energy deficit.

If you are diagnosed as suffering from low blood sugar, the condition can often be corrected by a diet free of refined carbohydrates (table sugar and sweets) and rich in complex carbohydrates, as well as foods high in magnesium and zinc, which play a role in regulating the function of the pancreas. In addition, eating a meal containing protein, especially beans, or a nutritious snack every two to three hours helps to maintain blood sugar at a constant level and therefore keep the release of insulin to a healthy level.

MIGRAINE AND OTHER HEADACHES

There are many types and causes of headache. If you have severe or persistent attacks, you should seek professional advice.

Migraines and other headaches can sometimes be induced by intolerance to specific foods, particularly those that contain high levels of amine compounds. Examples are coffee, chocolate, cheese, oranges, and red wine. It is important to determine what foods trigger your headaches by keeping a food diary (see page 21) and avoid these.

Low blood sugar levels can also trigger headaches, so make sure that you maintain a steady level of blood sugar by eating regular and nutritious meals.

Avoiding a hangover

Headaches that follow an overindulgence in food or drink are likely to be part of a hangover. If you are embarking on a celebration that will involve alcohol, a few simple measures can reduce the risk of unpleasant aftereffects. The most effective approach is to limit your consumption of alcohol to no more than one or two drinks and follow them with plenty of water. (If you are a woman, remember that your liver is less efficient at breaking down alcohol than that of a man, so your capacity for drinking is less.) For most people the pleasure of drinking diminishes rapidly after two or three drinks anyway.

Do not drink on an empty stomach, but bear in mind that food slows down the rate of clearance of alcohol from the blood, so eat moderately before drinking.

Do not mix your drinks, especially those derived from grapes (wine) and grains (beer and spirits like whisky). Drink plenty of water during and after celebrations to minimize the dehydration that will be brought about by the alcohol.

More significant than a hangover is the fact that regular high alcohol intake can lead to more serious disorders like cirrhosis of the liver, so it is best to make a practice of stopping after one or two social drinks.

JET LAG

Traveling rapidly between different time zones on long-distance flights disturbs your body rhythms and routines. Your bowel, bladder, and sleeping pattern can all be disrupted for some days after a long flight, and there is also some evidence for a depression of the immune function, making you more susceptible to infections. Other symptoms, such as tiredness and poor concentration, are common after long-distance travel, particularly at times when you would have been sleeping at home.

For a few days before a long flight, include in your diet plenty of vegetables, fruits, and whole grains, which will provide protective minerals and trace elements plus vitamins A, C, and E, the antioxidant nutrients that support immune function. Eat only a moderate amount of protein-rich foods because the metabolism of large amounts of protein overloads the liver and kidneys, which are important in coping with the strain of travel on the body. It may help to eat sunflower and sesame seeds during your flight; these provide essential fatty acids that regulate stress hormones.

To arrive at your destination feeling as fresh as possible, follow the tips below for gradually rearranging your mealtimes and sleeping routine.

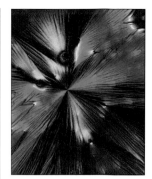

VITAMIN C
The colored micrograph image above shows vitamin C. Tests have confirmed that consuming vitamin C-rich foods and drinks during celebrations may help your body eliminate alcohol more quickly.

AVOIDING JET LAG

You can help your body adapt more readily to time changes and travel stress by introducing a few changes in dietary habits and sleeping routine a few days in advance of traveling. These adjustments will shorten the time that your body needs to get used to a new time zone.

A few days before your journey, start changing your habits to fit the time zone of your destination. If traveling east, this means rising and retiring earlier.

Avoid large rich meals for a few days before your flight and eat lots of fresh fruits and vegetables to build up levels of antioxidant nutrients.

Try to sleep as much as possible, especially at times when your destination is in darkness.

On your flight, adjust your eating habits to those of your destination time. If an in-flight meal is offered at a time when you would be sleeping at your destination, skip it.

Avoid alcoholic drinks and coffee, which will increase dehydration, but take plenty of other fluids (water, fruit juices, and herbal teas) to prevent this. Avoid fizzy drinks, which can make you feel bloated on a flight.

MOUTH, EYE, AND EAR DISORDERS

Problems with the mouth, eyes, and ears are commonplace and affect everyone at some time. Dietary measures are very effective at preventing many of these problems and relieving others.

Mouth, eye, and ear disorders are among the most aggravating of health problems because they affect some of our most frequently used organs. A balanced diet plays an essential part in preventing and relieving these problems before they become debilitating.

MOUTH PROBLEMS

As an active region of the mucous tissue at the start of the digestive and respiratory tracts, the mouth and its constituent parts reflect very much what is going on further down in both lungs and stomach.

Problems with mucus may be worsened by dairy products. Incorporating onions, garlic, and ginger in your cooking will help counteract mucus and stimulate digestive activities at the same time. A raw-food diet or a cleansing program may also help.

Mouth ulcers

Ulcers, which may appear on the tongue or gums or in the cheeks, are caused by the *Herpes simplex* virus. It multiplies when immunity is low, and sugars in the diet are believed to encourage adhesion of the virus to cell walls. If you have mouth ulcers, avoid foods high in sugar and build your immunity with foods high in antioxidants.

Research has shown that the amino acid lysine has an antiviral quality that may cause its aggressive reaction with arginine, another amino acid. If you have recurrent mouth ulcers, it may be helpful to increase lysine-rich foods, such as fish, brewer's yeast, and cheese, and reduce those with a higher ratio of arginine, such as sunflower seeds, whole grains, and meat.

Bad breath (halitosis)

There are many possible causes of bad breath. Food intolerance, in which incomplete digestion leads to fermentation in the stomach or intestines, is one. Constipation, which reduces the rate of elimination of putrefactive compounds, is another. Both can give rise to gases from the fermentation of compounds and lead to halitosis.

Chronic catarrh (inflamation of mucuous membranes) in sinuses or bronchial tubes may cause an unpleasant odor or taste in the mouth. Also, diabetes can cause a sickly sweet odor on the breath. A diet high in refined carbohydrates, such as sugar or white flour, is another possible contender. Frequent intake of aromatic drinks like tea, coffee, and alcohol can also create offensive breath.

When fasting, some patients start to draw on body reserves in a process known as ketosis. This breakdown of protein compounds is another known cause of halitosis.

SAGE RELIEF

The culinary herb sage (*Salvia officinalis*) has soothing antiseptic and antibiotic properties. (*Salvia* comes from a Latin word meaning "to heal.") To prepare a weak infusion, steep 2 teaspoons of chopped fresh leaves or 1 teaspoon of dried for about 10 minutes in a cup of boiling water, then strain. Use the tea as a gargle to ease a sore throat or mouth ulcers or as a mouth rinse to freshen the breath.

Sage should be avoided by pregnant women, although small amounts as a flavoring in cooking are considered safe.

A substance in sage oil, called thujone, can be toxic. Undiluted sage oil should not be taken internally nor applied to the skin. Sage extracts should also be used with caution.

SAGE (red variety shown) The pungent leaves of this herb have a long history of relieving problems of the mouth and throat.

Halitosis can also be a side effect of gum disease and tooth decay (see below). Once the underlying cause has been treated, the bad breath should disappear. Meanwhile, suck or chew lemon slices, parsley, or peppermint to help freshen the breath.

Gum disease

Food particles trapped between the teeth and gums may lead to increased bacterial activity and gum disease. Regular brushing and flossing can help reduce this.

Gum disease can sometimes be a consequence of poor digestion. A short cleansing or detoxification diet program can help to reduce the fermentation that takes place in the mouth or stomach. Follow this with raw vegetables and fruit in conjunction with a balanced diet. To protect your gums, avoid sugary foods and drinks.

Tooth decay

Regular brushing and flossing are certainly a vital part of preventing tooth decay. Bacteria in the mouth can form a sticky film, called plaque, over the surface of teeth. Bacteria in the plaque break down the sugars and starches in food and turn them into acids. Unless plaque is regularly removed, the acids it produces dissolve tooth enamel and cause decay. It is especially important to brush teeth right after eating sticky foods, such as dried apricots and peanut butter.

The part that diet plays in preventing tooth decay is to build strong teeth and gums through good nutrition. Foods rich in calcium and phosphorus are especially important; these include not only dairy products but also green leafy vegetables,

Chewing on crisp raw foods like cauliflower, peppers, and apples provides not only necessary nutrients but also exercise, which strengthens teeth and gums, and an increase in saliva, which reduces bacteria.

Another aid in preventing tooth decay is tea, which helps teeth resist acid. The substances in tea thought to provide this benefit are tannin, catechin, caffeine, and tocopherol. The effects are even better when tea is made with water that contains fluoride.

EYE PROBLEMS

Eyes not only register the world around us but also receive natural light, which is believed to be important for glandular health and immunity. Diseases of the eye,

BULGUR WITH TOFU AND RED PEPPER

This delicious dish is rich in vitamins A and C from the spinach and the peppers. Both of these antioxidants are known to help prevent cataracts.

100 g/4 oz coarse or medium bulgur
1 tbsp sunflower oil
2 cloves garlic, peeled and finely crushed
1 tsp ground cumin
1 medium red bell pepper, seeded and cut into strips
2 tbsp vinegar
2 tbsp water
225 g/8 oz fresh spinach, washed, stemmed, and cut into strips
freshly ground black pepper and salt to taste
225 g/8 oz firm tofu, cut into cubes

- Rinse the bulgur in a colander under cold running water. Put it in a large bowl, cover it with cold water, and leave it to soak for at least an hour; then drain off the water.
- Heat the oil in a large skillet over medium heat and cook the garlic, stirring it constantly, for a few seconds or until soft.
- Add the cumin and bell pepper, cover the pan, and cook for 5 minutes. Add the drained bulgur, the vinegar, and water to the pan and cook, uncovered, for 5 minutes or until the bulgur is nearly soft, stirring frequently.
- Add the spinach and stir thoroughly until it is well mixed with the other ingredients. Season with the pepper and salt.
- Add the tofu, then cover the pan and simmer for 5 minutes or until the tofu is heated through.

Serves 4

such as glaucoma and cataracts, can completely remove the capacity for sight. Although the evidence for beneficial nutritional measures in this area is inconclusive, there are some proven dietary facts. The progress of glaucoma may be delayed by a diet low in salt, caffeine, and alcohol, while vitamins A, B_2, C, and E are believed to have some protective effects against many eye disorders.

Cataract, a degenerative condition that causes the lens of the eye to become opaque, is possibly caused by an obstruction of the normal routes of nourishment to the eye. There is a possibility that changes in blood sugar levels may play a part because diabetics are prone to the condition. Vitamins A, C, and E are reported to be beneficial in delaying development of the condition. Adequate riboflavin (vitamin B_2) is also important. Increase your intake of orange vegetables and leafy greens for vitamin A; citrus fruits, kiwifruit, sweet peppers, and cruciferous vegetables for vitamin C; wheat germ and vegetable oils for vitamin E; and

Kidney energy
In Chinese medicine the energy of the kidneys is regarded as nourishing the ears. Kidney energy is sustained by "warming" foods, so to help prevent hearing loss, Chinese therapists recommend eating more sesame seeds, tofu, walnuts, eggs, and ginger.

include more meat, poultry, fish, eggs, milk products, and fortified cereals for riboflavin.

Night blindness

Poor vision in dim light or in the dark may be the first sign of a vitamin A deficiency. Vitamin A is necessary for the formation of visual purple, a pigment in the retina that enables the eye to adjust from bright to dark conditions. Foods rich in vitamin A include carrots and other orange vegetables, sweet red peppers, spinach and other dark leafy greens, liver, and whole-milk products. Raw vegetables and their juices can be beneficial, but lightly cooked vegetables are often a better source of vitamin A.

The trace element zinc, found in shellfish, particularly oysters, is also involved in the activity of vitamin A in the retina. This means that for you to benefit as much as possible from the vitamin A in your diet, you must also take in a reasonable amount

of zinc-rich foods. Some members of the family of B vitamins—riboflavin (B_2), thiamine (B_1), and niacin (B_3)—are also necessary. These vitamins are present in whole grains, wheat germ, brewer's yeast and organ meats, such as liver.

EAR PROBLEMS

Because degenerative hearing loss comes to many people as they age, it is not uncommon for people to simply accept that their hearing is fading. In fact, hearing loss may be caused by easily remedied disorders, such as an excessive mucus buildup (catarrh).

Catarrh from unresolved nasal and sinus disorders can thicken and partially block the eustachian tube, which connects the middle ear and throat. This impairs transmission of sound waves to the inner ear. To overcome chronic catarrh, eat plenty of garlic and onions and vitamin C–rich foods, such as sweet peppers and broccoli.

Intermittent hearing loss has been linked to low blood-sugar levels. The adrenaline increase induced by low blood sugar causes a constriction of the blood vessels in the ear. In 1975 two doctors, E. J. Gorselin and P. Yanik, writing in the *Journal of the American Audiological Society*, reported that a study of 90 patients with hearing loss showed that 58 percent had reactive hypoglycemia. Avoiding sugary foods and making other changes in the diet may therefore be of benefit (see page 96).

Tinnitus and Ménière's disease

Noises in the ears (tinnitus)—usually high-pitched ringing or whistles or low-pitched hisses—are believed to be associated with a disturbance of blood flow in the inner ear. Improving blood viscosity by reducing saturated fat and cholesterol in the diet may help relieve the condition and also prevent buildup of atherosclerotic plaque in the ears, which can lead to hearing loss.

Ménière's disease, characterized by dizziness, vertigo, and nausea, is caused by excessive fluid in the inner ear. Because too much salt in the diet can increase fluid retention by the body, doctors advise a low-salt diet to prevent buildup of inner ear fluid and diuretics to rid the body of fluid that has already accumulated. Ginger tea or crystallized ginger can help relieve the nausea.

VEGETABLE MÉLANGE WITH CORIANDER

Tomatoes are a useful source of beta carotene, which will boost your levels of vitamin A and help relieve tinnitus. Eating this vegetable dish on a bed of brown rice or millet will ensure that you also have a healthy intake of magnesium.

2 tbsp olive oil
2 cloves garlic, peeled and crushed
1 onion, peeled and chopped
8 button mushrooms, washed
100 g/4 oz cauliflower florets, washed
2 stalks celery, washed and chopped
400 g/14 oz can tomatoes, chopped
6 coriander seeds
1 bouquet garni (parsley and thyme sprigs and 1 bay leaf tied in a bunch)
4 tbsp dry white wine
1 tbsp green peppercorns
salt to taste
fresh cilantro (coriander leaves) for garnish

■ Heat the oil in a large skillet over moderate heat, add the garlic, and cook for 2 minutes but do not brown. Stir in the onion, mushrooms, cauliflower, and celery.
■ Add the tomatoes and bring to a boil. Add the coriander seeds, bouquet garni, wine, peppercorns, and salt. Simmer, uncovered, for 15 to 20 minutes or until the vegetables are just tender and the liquid has been reduced.
■ Discard the bouquet garni; spoon vegetables into a serving dish and garnish with the cilantro. Serve with boiled or steamed millet or brown rice.

Serves 4

RESPIRATORY DISORDERS

The respiratory system includes the upper airways (nose and throat), the lungs, and the tubes that join them. All of these may be affected by allergens, infections, and intolerance to foods.

When your respiratory system is adversely affected by an external influence, whether it be a virus, bacteria, an allergen such as pollen, or a contaminant in the air, like a pesticide, the delicate and sensitive mucous membranes in your nose and throat may swell and itch and have involuntary spasms, more commonly known as coughs and sneezes.

Although some respiratory disorders are related to food allergies or intolerance and will respond well to dietary changes, when the disorder results from an infection, the first line of dietary defense must be one that boosts the immune system with nutrient-rich foods and helps to aid recovery.

COLDS

The common cold is an inflammation of the mucous membranes in the nose and throat, caused by any of more than 200 known viruses. Colds commonly occur during the winter months, possibly because this is a time when people group together indoors, thus making it easier for viruses to spread.

When treating a cold with food, the primary aims are to boost the immune system, thus helping it fight the infection, and to reduce mucus, which builds up because of the inflamed membranes. Mucus puts pressure on the membranes, and when it becomes very thick, it can cause painful blockages and breathing difficulties.

TREATMENT FOR COLDS AND COUGHS

From the moment a cold or cough begins, it is important to give your body as much assistance as you can to support its ability to fight back. This program, most effective if used for three days, will boost your intake of vitamin-rich foods and help lessen the unpleasant effects of the cough or cold.

 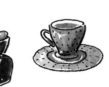 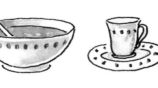 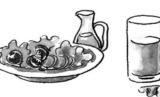

ON RISING
Hot lemon and honey or cider vinegar and honey—1 teaspoon of each in a cup of hot water. You can add chopped fresh ginger too.

BREAKFAST
Fresh fruit mixture, such as grapes, apples, bananas, peaches, and oranges.

MIDMORNING
Herbal tea, fruit juice, or hot bouillon.

LUNCH
Two or three steamed vegetables, a vegetable soup, or a mixed vegetable stew. Flavor with miso (fermented soy bean paste) if desired.

AFTERNOON
Same as for midmorning.

DINNER
Mixed raw salad, including onions or garlic, with dressing based on cider vinegar and olive oil or sunflower oil. (Lunch and dinner menus may be switched if you prefer.)

BEFORE BED
Hot lemon and honey or ginger tea.

Prevent a cold

The common cold is caused by a virus. You can reduce your susceptibility to catching a cold and aid recovery from one by strengthening your immune system with dietary measures. Foods rich in vitamins C and A are particularly beneficial.

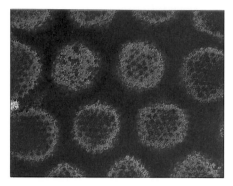

THE COLD VIRUS
More than 200 viruses are known to cause the symptoms of a common cold; a microscopic image of one is shown above. The vast majority of these viruses are passed between people through the air.

DEFICIENCY PREVENTION

Even mild vitamin and mineral deficiencies, which may not show up in blood tests, can reduce your immune system's effectiveness, particularly when you are under stress or suffering from a cold. The best way to prevent such deficiencies

Food itself cannot stop an infection; only the body's defenses can combat germs effectively. The infection must run its course until the immune system has it under control. In the meantime, it can help to stay warm, drink hot liquids, and eat plenty of fruit.

Deficiencies of zinc, selenium, and vitamins A and C have all been shown to deplete the immune system.

is to eat a wide variety of foods that contain the full range of nutrients you need and as little as possible of refined sugar and milled cereals and rice. Grains can lose 90 percent or more of essential minerals like zinc during the refining process.

Vitamin A is made in the body from beta carotene, found in orange and green vegetables, such as carrots and peppers. Citrus fruits and peppers are good sources of vitamin C, and zinc is abundant in oysters, legumes, shellfish, meat, whole grains, and sunflower seeds. For selenium-rich foods, eat Brazil nuts, seafood, eggs, meat, whole grains, and legumes.

From ancient times to the present, garlic has been used to fight colds. If you can tolerate it, infuse fresh garlic in hot water and drink the brew twice daily until your cold is gone. To get rid of the resulting bad breath, chew fresh parsley.

VITAMIN C SUPPLEMENTS
Taking vitamin C supplements cannot stop a cold but will help you fight one (1,000 mg per day is usually effective). The vitamin helps relieve symptoms and then fights the infection. If you stop the supplements too soon, your cold may return with a vengeance. Once symptoms are gone, however, you should taper off the vitamin C because an excess can cause diarrhea.

Although there is concern that high doses of vitamin C may cause kidney stones, so far there has been no conclusive evidence to support this notion.

FEED A COLD AND STARVE A FEVER

This old adage may be true to some extent. If you have a cold, it is important to increase your intake of nutrient-rich foods to help your body

fight the infection. For a fever, which can cause nausea and loss of appetite, it may be best to consume only small amounts of food and lots of liquids.

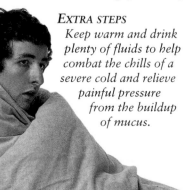

EXTRA STEPS
Keep warm and drink plenty of fluids to help combat the chills of a severe cold and relieve painful pressure from the buildup of mucus.

FOOD TO FIGHT COLDS
A small bowl of warming vitamin C-rich soup, such as tomato and orange, is an ideal dish for a person suffering a cold.

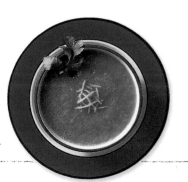

Fighting the infection

It is important to eat foods containing vitamin C, the B vitamins, and zinc, which will help the immune system to fight off infection. During a severe cold, eat a lot of fresh fruit for two days, followed by salads and vegetable stews for two to three days more; these are easily digested sources of vitamins and minerals. Include pumpkin seeds in your salads for their zinc content. Eat oranges with the pith still on; this is rich in the bioflavonoid complex related to vitamin C. (Bioflavonoid compounds are believed to protect mucous membranes.)

Breaking down the mucus

For colds and chest problems with large amounts of mucus, reduce dairy products and starchy foods and eat plenty of fresh fruits and vegetables. In addition, sip chicken soup. Studies have shown that it eases nasal congestion better than hot water or tea.

COUGHS

Coughs have many variations, from the intense, hacking type caused by a chest infection to the dry, tickling variety caused by a sore throat. Although a cough can be a sign of other, more serious disorders, short-term remedies for minor infections and irritations can be very effective.

If the cough is caused by an infection, the immune system needs to be strengthened to help fight the infection. This can be achieved either by increasing your intake of foods that build up the immune system (see page 36) or by cutting down on the foods that may weaken it, especially those that are high in sugar.

Some coughs are exacerbated by dairy products, particularly milk. Environmental irritants, such as cigarette smoke and traffic fumes, may also have a negative effect. If the cough is due to an allergic reaction, it is important to identify the allergen to which you are reacting. If the allergen is a food,

---

DID YOU KNOW?

A raw onion, chopped and mixed with a spoonful of honey, is a reliable remedy for a tight, tickly cough. The combination helps expel mucus from the chest. Chew the mixture two or three times a day, followed by a parsley sprig to prevent bad breath.

GAZPACHO SOUP

Rich in vitamin C and other important nutrients, this tasty and spicy soup is ideal for someone suffering with a cold.

1.25 kg/2½ lb ripe tomatoes, roughly chopped
2 medium onions, peeled and chopped
2 green bell peppers, seeded and chopped
1 large cucumber, chopped
3 tbsp red wine vinegar or tarragon vinegar
2 tbsp olive oil
½ tsp sugar
2 cloves garlic, peeled and crushed
350 ml/1½ cups tomato juice
freshly ground black pepper and salt to taste

■ Reserve a little of each chopped vegetable to use as a garnish. Place the remaining vegetables in a food processor or blender.
■ Add the vinegar, olive oil, sugar, garlic, and tomato juice and blend until almost smooth. Season with pepper and salt. If you prefer a smoother soup, strain it through a fine sieve.
■ Transfer the soup to a large bowl, cover, and chill well. Place the garnish vegetables in a separate bowl, cover, and chill.
■ Divide the soup evenly among six bowls and top each serving with some of the reserved vegetables.
Serves 6

you should try to remove it from your diet as soon as possible.

If a cough is persistent or becomes worse with dietary treatment, it is very important to seek medical advice.

BRONCHITIS

Bronchitis, which may be caused either by a virus or by bacteria, can be a chronic and often severe pulmonary infection. Characterized by congestion and inflammation of the bronchial tubes, with coughing and a lot of mucus, outbreaks of bronchitis are prevalent during the winter months, especially among the elderly. Chest pain often accompanies the symptoms, but any attendant fever is usually mild.

If you suffer from persistent colds or chest complaints, it is wise to have a checkup and get some professional advice on strengthening your immune system, especially if there is any hint of chronic bronchitis developing.

As with a severe cold, if you suffer from bronchitis, follow the dietary guidelines set out above. Futhermore, you should avoid foods that are high in refined sugar and

WINTER VEGETABLE CASSEROLE

The onions and garlic in this casserole will help break down mucus, and the vitamin C and beta carotene from the fresh vegetables will help the immune system fight the infection that has caused a cold or bronchitis.

1 tbsp sunflower oil
2 large onions, roughly chopped
2 leeks, sliced
3 cloves garlic, peeled and finely chopped
3 potatoes, cubed
3 carrots, peeled and cubed
1 small rutabaga, peeled and cubed
1 sweet potato, peeled and cubed
900 ml/3½ cups water or vegetable stock
1 tsp minced fresh oregano or 2 tsp dried leaves
1 tsp minced fresh thyme or 2 tsp dried leaves
2 small zucchini, cut in chunks
freshly ground black pepper and salt to taste
chopped fresh parsley for garnish

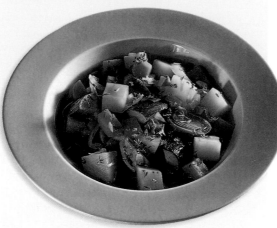

■ Heat the oil in a large heavy saucepan or stockpot over medium heat. Add the onions, leeks, and garlic and cook until softened. Add the cubed vegetables, the water or stock, oregano, and thyme and stir well.
■ Bring to a boil, then cover and simmer for 30 minutes or until the vegetables are tender. Add the zucchini. Season with pepper and salt.
■ Simmer over medium heat for 5 minutes or until the zucchini is tender. Spoon into bowls and sprinkle each serving with the parsley.
Serves 4

THE ASTHMATIC REACTION

When an asthma attack occurs, the bronchioles, the tubes that carry air into the lungs, become constricted. This constriction causes the characteristic wheezing of asthma.

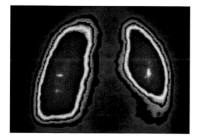

HEALTHY LUNGS
The red areas in the photo above show the densest areas of air in the main chambers of the lungs.

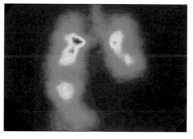

ASTHMATIC LUNGS
The yellow areas, above, show asthmatic obstruction; the left lung is more congested than the right.

---

drink plenty of fluids every day. These measures should help your immune system begin to fight off the infection.

ASTHMA

The difficulty in breathing and the wheezes of asthma are caused by obstruction of the airways by either spasmodic narrowing of the bronchial tubes or their blockage with excessive mucus. Asthmatics always need medical treatment, but appropriate environmental and dietary measures can do much to alleviate the problems.

Bronchial spasm is often caused by allergic sensitivity to substances that are breathed in, such as pollen, house dust, mites, or molds, and occasionally to foods, such as eggs, shellfish, or peanuts. Cow's milk may also be a factor in asthma, either because it acts as an allergen or because it stimulates mucus production.

In one long-term study a vegan diet (one that excludes all animal products) helped relieve asthma to some degree in 23 out of 25 patients. The doctor who conducted the research suggested that arachidonic acid, found in meat and dairy foods, increases inflammatory substances in the body called leukotrienes, which trigger attacks.

Other studies have shown that low blood sugar and low levels of vitamin C and magnesium are also associated with higher levels of histamine, an inflammatory substance that can contribute to asthma inflammation. Allergic individuals need to stabilize their energy levels and eat vitamin C-rich foods.

Some asthmatics are allergic to additives, particularly the sulfite compounds found in fruit juices, wine, and dried fruit. People who are sensitive should avoid them.

Caffeine contains theophylline (now included in asthma drugs), which is a bronchodilator—that is, it widens the airways constricted during an asthma attack. In a study done in 1986, it was discovered that a single cup of brewed coffee produced as much as a 15 percent increase in breathing capacity. However, excessive caffeine has side effects, such as heart palpitations and headaches, and should never be used when a patient is taking antispasmodic drugs that contain theophylline.

Sulfur compounds in onions have an antiflammatory effect. Raw onions can likely be helpful in both preventing and reducing the inflammation of an asthma attack.

Digestive Disorders

A stomach upset may be caused by bacteria in foods, but the problem can also lie with the digestive process itself. Improving your digestion can be a first step to improving your health.

The stomach and intestines, together with the liver, gallbladder, and pancreas, are the powerhouse of the body. Because they process everything we eat or drink to provide energy for activity, growth, and repair, changes in diet are an essential part of a healing program for digestive disorders.

CELIAC DISEASE

The intestinal disorder called celiac disease is characterized by diarrhea, colic, abdominal bloating, and in children, poor growth. It tends to run in families and is caused by an intolerance to gliadin, part of the protein gluten, found in wheat, oats, barley, and rye. Celiacs must replace gluten-containing foods with others that have comparable amounts of complex carbohydrates, fiber, vitamins, and minerals. Rice, corn, and potatoes are alternative sources of carbohydrate and fiber. Rice, soy, corn, and potato flours are available for making bread.

Many emulsifiers and stabilizers, found in such processed foods as lunch meats, chocolate drinks, and pudding mixes, are made from gluten. Celiacs should avoid these and products that list ingredients like vegetable gum or vegetable protein, hydrolyzed vegetable protein, and malt.

Because gluten damages the lining of the small intestine in celiacs, thus preventing efficient absorption of nutrients, deficiencies, particularly of iron, folic acid, vitamin B_{12}, and the fat-soluble vitamins, A, D, E, and K, often occur in celiac patients. They should eat plenty of fruits, green vegetables, and legumes for their vitamin and mineral content, as well as their fiber. Seeds, such as sunflower and pumpkin, will provide iron and essential fatty acids to protect against inflammation of the intestinal lining. Tahini (ground sesame seeds) is rich in calcium and can be used for salad dressings and sauces.

The damage to their intestines makes many celiacs intolerant to dairy products. They can use calcium-enriched soy milk instead. Celiac-induced diarrhea also causes considerable loss of healthy bacteria from the intestines, but these can be replaced to some extent by fermented foods, such as yogurt with live cultures and sauerkraut.

CONSTIPATION

Difficulty in passing stools, infrequency of stools, and small hard feces are all forms of constipation. Stress may bring on an occasional bout of constipation, so can eating something you're not used to. Regular or persistent constipation is often caused by a loss of tone in the walls of the intestines as a result of insufficient fiber. Everyone should have 20 to 35 grams of fiber a day; many people consume no more than 12.

Magnesium may also be a factor in long-term constipation because a deficiency in this mineral causes muscle spasms that prevent the bowels from working properly. Magnesium is found in whole-grain cereals, legumes, leafy green vegetables, and eggs.

There are two kinds of fiber: insoluble, found primarily in bran, nuts, whole grains, and fruit and vegetable skins; and soluble, contained in the flesh of many fruits and

SUNFLOWER AND PUMPKIN SEEDS
A handful of these seeds each day can boost iron in celiac sufferers and also protect them against inflammation of the intestinal lining.

105

THE DIGESTIVE SYSTEM

Each element of food is affected by specific enzymes that come into play at various stages of the digestive process and help the body to reap the highest benefits from food.

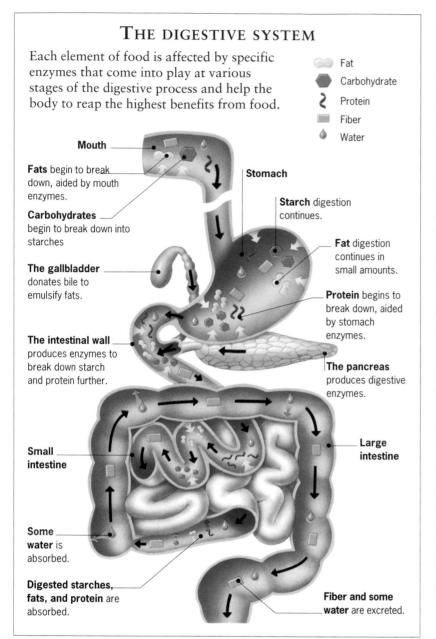

- 🍥 Fat
- ⬡ Carbohydrate
- 2 Protein
- ▭ Fiber
- 💧 Water

Mouth

Fats begin to break down, aided by mouth enzymes.

Carbohydrates begin to break down into starches

The gallbladder donates bile to emulsify fats.

The intestinal wall produces enzymes to break down starch and protein further.

Small intestine

Some water is absorbed.

Digested starches, fats, and protein are absorbed.

Stomach

Starch digestion continues.

Fat digestion continues in small amounts.

Protein begins to break down, aided by stomach enzymes.

The pancreas produces digestive enzymes.

Large intestine

Fiber and some water are excreted.

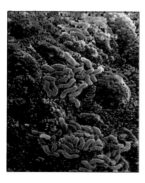

*HEALTHY GUT BACTERIA
The purple bacteria, above, occur naturally in the gut and help the body break down food.*

vegetables, nuts, and legumes. The insoluble type passes through the digestive tract largely unchanged and is important because it gives bulk to the stools. Soluble fiber dissolves and becomes sticky.

Because fiber absorbs a great deal of water, any increase in fiber must be accompanied by a similar increase in fluid intake. Drink fresh fruit and vegetable juices and at least a quart of water every day.

DIARRHEA

Short bouts of diarrhea can be caused by eating too much fresh or dried fruit, too many spicy foods, or a food you are not used to. This type of diarrhea will last only until the body has rid itself of that particular food. Food contaminated with harmful bacteria, high and prolonged levels of stress, and too many stimulants like caffeine are other causes. An attack of diarrhea can also follow a course of antibiotics, which disturb the healthy bacteria in the large intestine. Eating fermented products, such as yogurt and tofu, may help replenish them.

Diarrhea over a longer period may be due to gastroenteritis or a chronic bowel disorder such as celiac disease (see page 105) or colitis. Also, incomplete digestion of certain foods because of enzyme deficiencies may result in undigested food fermenting in the intestines and causing irritation that can lead to diarrhea and flatulence.

If diarrhea lasts for more than two days, it can help to fast for 24 hours, drinking only fresh apple, carrot, or diluted pineapple juice and mineral water to allow the digestive system to clear away the undigested food. It's important to drink at least six glasses of water a day to counter dehydration caused by diarrhea. Some doctors also advise having a sports drink to replace the electrolytes (sodium and potassium) lost in diarrhea.

On the second day eat a little yogurt with live cultures for breakfast and top it with grated or puréed apple. Introduce steamed rice or millet the next day as you build up to a normal diet. Eat pectin-rich foods, such as apples and pears (best grated raw, but stewed is also fine), because pectin helps bacteria to multiply. Another time-tested approach is to follow the BRAT diet—banana, rice, applesauce, and toast.

COLITIS

Colitis is a chronic inflammation of the large intestine and rectum, characterized by abdominal cramps, persistent diarrhea, rectal bleeding, fever, and weight loss. It should always be investigated by a doctor. During a flare-up a bland, low-fiber diet is recommended, with no raw vegetables or fruits, nuts, seeds, or bran. Colitis sufferers

DID YOU KNOW?
Rice gruel or water from boiled rice is a traditional remedy in developing countries. It is used for countering the dehydration caused by chronic diarrhea and is known to be effective.

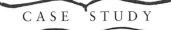
A Celiac Sufferer

The dietary needs of the celiac patient are more specific than those of people who have other digestive disorders. After what might be years of unidentified digestive problems, an accurate diagnosis and well-planned diet and lifestyle can make a big difference in the quality of life for a celiac sufferer.

At the age of 28, Paula is an assistant manager in the lingerie department of a large store, but at busy times her erratic bowels cause her both discomfort and embarrassment. Her personnel record shows that she has taken a lot of sick leave, and she believes that her job is taking a toll on her health. She is reluctant to go out socially, for fear of being unable to find a restroom should the need arise suddenly, so she often spends evenings alone.

Paula has been subject to stomach troubles and has had difficulty putting on weight for a few years now. She is becoming increasingly tired and listless and has decided to get to the root of her problem. It has become a threat to her health, career, and social life.

WHAT SHOULD PAULA DO?

Paula's family doctor referred her to a specialist in gastroenterology, who discovered that she is suffering from a gluten sensitivity known as celiac disease. This hereditary disorder, in which a person is unable to absorb gluten, a protein in wheat, barley, rye, and oats, slowly destroys the lining of the intestines. It causes digestive disturbances and prevents absorption of nutrients.

Paula was then sent to a dietitian, who gave her a list of gluten-containing foods that she must avoid in any form and suggested healthy alternatives. She was also given information on a suitable diet and advised to take vitamin and mineral supplements until her system recovers from nutritional deficiencies.

Action Plan

EATING HABITS
Check food labels and menus in restaurants for ingredients that contain gluten. For more information, contact the National Digestive Diseases Information Clearinghouse in Bethesda, Maryland.

DIET
Eat plenty of cooked vegetables and vegetable soups. Start each meal with a little grated apple or carrot to introduce raw fiber.

STRESS
Join a yoga class and learn to relax and breathe correctly in order to reduce the levels of anxiety experienced at work.

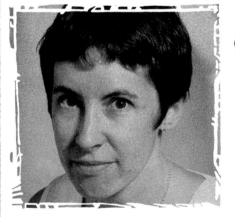

STRESS
Stressful situations can cause the rhythmical contractions of the intestines to speed up, leading to diarrhea.

EATING HABITS
Avoiding all foods that contain gluten is essential. Dairy products may also be a problem for sensitive and damaged intestinal membranes.

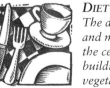

DIET
The depleted vitamin and mineral levels of the celiac patient need building up with vegetables and fruits. These also provide fiber for normal intestinal function.

HOW THINGS TURNED OUT FOR PAULA

Within a few weeks of following a gluten-free diet, Paula was having fewer digestive problems. As she gained confidence, her social life improved, and as her vitality increased, she felt able to do more exercise and tackle her work with new energy. Paula found a weekly yoga class that complemented the demands of her work, and her job became a pleasurable challenge rather than a drudge. She was promoted within six months.

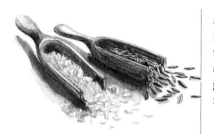

DIVERTICULOSIS AND FIBER
Fiber-rich foods, such as whole-grain cereals, help to strengthen the weakened bowel of someone who suffers with diverticulosis.

INCOMPATIBLE FOODS
Certain foods when eaten together are incompatible in some people. High-protein foods, like meat and eggs, and starches, such as the flour in a pie crust, are considered by some to be the main culprits. For example, a roast beef sandwich or chicken pot pie may cause terrible discomfort and bloating. If you suffer similarly, try eating your protein, starches, and even fruit, separately. A gap of four hours is usually enough.

also need to be especially careful about maintaining a well-balanced diet because they are prone to deficiencies, especially anemia. Liver, spinach and other dark leafy greens, dried beans, and fortified cereals are rich in iron to combat anemia.

DIVERTICULOSIS

A lack of adequate fiber in the diet can lead to a weakness of the muscular walls of the intestines in susceptible individuals. Diverticula, or pouches, may develop in the walls, and these often harbor fecal matter, which can cause diarrhea, constipation, abdominal pain, and bloating. If the pouches become inflamed or infected, diverticulosis may turn into diverticulitis, which frequently requires medical treatment with antibiotics and a bland diet of puréed cooked foods; sometimes surgery is needed.

Foods to relieve this condition are those rich in fiber: whole-grain cereals, vegetables, legumes, and fruits. Spicy foods, nuts, and seeds should be avoided.

FLATULENCE

Gas is often a normal consequence of eating some otherwise healthy foods, including beans, broccoli, and cabbage. It may also occur as a symptom of certain digestive disorders, like constipation, irritable bowel syndrome, or deficiencies of certain enzymes, such as those for digesting protein (common in the elderly). An enzyme deficiency can result in undigested food passing into the intestines, where it ferments. Lactose intolerance can also cause flatulence.

To curb flatulence, avoid foods that cause you great discomfort. For instance, if you have an intolerance to lactose, avoid dairy foods (some yogurts and cheeses may be tolerated because their bacteria break down lactose). When you are feeling bloated, try eating fresh pineapple or papaya, which contain natural enzymes that can help to relieve flatulence. Include plenty of fiber in the diet; it ensures regular bowel action, so that flatulence has little opportunity to build up. Certain herbs called carminatives (see page 80) also help to reduce gas.

Many sufferers find that gastro-

intestinal bloating and flatulence are reduced when they avoid food combinations that can be incompatible, such as starch (bread, rice, cereals, potatoes, and pastry) with protein (fish, eggs, and meat), or fruit after a meal or with starch. Incompatibility of certain foods is thought to occur because the digestion of starches requires alkaline enzymes, whereas that of protein requires acid enzymes.

IRRITABLE BOWEL SYNDROME

Frequent attacks of bloating and flatulence accompanied by pain and irregular bowel habits (sometimes constipation, sometimes diarrhea) are labeled irritable bowel syndrome (IBS) when there is no evidence that another digestive or inflammatory disorder is responsible for the symptoms. Several factors can be responsible for or contribute to the problem, including yeast overgrowth in the bowel, enzyme deficiency, and food intolerance. Major problem foods are wheat, cow's milk, sugar, tea, and coffee.

To overcome IBS you should first stop eating any foods that are known to cause bowel discomfort. At the same time, you should increase fiber in your diet to promote better movement of the intestinal walls and encourage beneficial bacteria to grow. This means eating more fruits and vegetables, whole-grain cereals, and oat bran (wheat bran is usually less tolerated).

If your condition does not improve with these measures, try treating the colon for overgrowth of yeast. This would require eliminating from your diet all foods that contain refined sugar because yeast thrives on sugar. Some people also find that wheat makes the condition worse. The live bacteria found in yogurt or acidophilus (bacteria) supplements can bring improvement, while a basic diet of fruit and vegetables and rice will allow the colon to recover.

ULCERS

Ulcers are sores that penetrate the underlying muscles of the digestive tract. Excessive smoking or intake of alcohol, continuous stress, and a diet that does not include enough fiber increase the danger of developing an ulcer. The heavy use of aspirin and other nonsteroidal anti-inflammatory drugs, which erode the stomach lining, is another risk factor. These create conditions in which *Helicobacter pylori*, the bacterium responsible for the condition, can thrive.

A gnawing, burning pain in the upper abdomen two or three hours after a meal is a typical symptom; it can usually be relieved by eating a little food. If you suspect that you have an ulcer, you should see a doctor right away. If the diagnosis is confirmed, you can try complementary dietary measures under the guidance of a dietitian, as well as conventional treatment.

In the early days after an ulcer has been diagnosed, your doctor may advise you to include more fiber—in the form of steamed vegetables and vegetable soups, brown rice or barley, and grated apples—in your diet, as much as 35 grams a day. Fiber helps strengthen the stomach lining.

A major healing food for ulcers is raw cabbage juice. Up to a quart a day is needed to achieve results, but it is very effective. Cabbage juice does have the unpleasant side effect of causing bloating and intestinal gas, but these usually diminish as the digestive system adjusts. Also, a gruel made with the powder of slippery elm bark is a particularly good healer of inflamed mucous membranes.

NAUSEA

Disturbances of the stomach, liver, or gallbladder can make you feel nauseated. Other forms of nausea include motion sickness, the side effects of chemotherapy for cancer, and the queasiness experienced in the early months of pregnancy.

For recurring nausea, as occurs during pregnancy, eat a savory snack, such as soda crackers, between meals and just before going to bed at night. This is particularly helpful if you suffer from low blood sugar, a common cause of nausea during pregnancy. Savory snacks may also help relieve nausea caused by digestive disturbances, but if the problem persists, you should see a doctor.

Ginger can help settle nausea, regardless of the cause. Sip ginger ale, eat candied ginger, add ginger slices to herbal tea, or prepare ginger tea by steeping a couple of slices of ginger in boiling water for 10 minutes. Taking ginger tablets before and during travel can prevent motion sickness as effectively as Dramamine, without the drowsiness sometimes caused by the drug.

DID YOU KNOW?

The bland diet once recommended for ulcer patients is no longer considered necessary, although it may help some people. It is important, however, to avoid foods that cause pain. Typical offenders are spicy dishes, caffeinated and alcoholic drinks, tomatoes, and chocolate.

BARLEY AND VEGETABLE SOUP

This delicious soup can soothe the discomfort of a stomach ulcer. And the fiber from its barley and vegetables will aid the growth of the stomach's protective mucous lining.

1.5 liters/6 cups chicken or vegetable stock
bouquet garni (parsley and thyme sprigs and 1 bay leaf, tied together)
75 g/3 oz pearl barley
25 g/1 tbsp margarine
3 carrots, peeled and sliced
3 stalks celery, sliced
1 large onion, peeled and chopped
225 g/8 oz mushrooms, washed and roughly chopped, including stems
1 tbsp lemon juice
freshly ground black pepper and salt to taste

■ Bring 600 ml/2½ cups of the stock to a boil. Add the bouquet garni and barley and simmer for 45 minutes.
■ Melt the margarine in a large saucepan over medium heat and cook the carrots, celery, and onion until the onion is soft. Add the cooked barley and remaining 840 ml/3½ cups of stock; simmer 10 minutes more.
■ Add the mushrooms and cook 5 minutes more. Remove the bouquet garni and add the lemon juice, pepper, and salt
Serves 4

CHILLED MELON AND YOGURT SOUP

This chilled, refreshing soup makes a delicious snack or light meal. It has the added attraction of providing quick relief from the discomfort of nausea.

1 large cantaloupe, halved and seeded
225 g/8 oz low-fat plain yogurt
3 tbsp lemon juice
1 tsp peeled and grated fresh ginger
2 tbsp chopped fresh mint

■ Using a soupspoon, scoop the flesh out of the melon and purée it in a food processor or blender. You can push it through a hard plastic strainer if you don't have one of these appliances.
■ Add the yogurt, lemon juice, and ginger. Mix well and then chill.
■ Spoon into bowls and top with the mint.
Serves 4

Diarrhea and constipation

Generally, diarrhea results from the bowel not absorbing enough fluid from the matter that passes through it, leaving the matter waterlogged; in constipation the bowel absorbs too much water, leaving the matter hard and difficult to move.

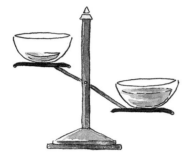

THE WATER BALANCE
An ideal situation is to have just the right amount of water passing from food matter into the bowel. Too much or too little can cause problems.

A persistent, unexplained change in bowel habits should be reported to your doctor because there could be a serious cause. Diarrhea may result from an infection (perhaps contracted on a trip); colitis or irritable bowel syndrome, often brought on by stress; an allergy or sensitivity to certain foods, such as onions, milk, and tomatoes; or bowel surgery.

FOODS FOR DIARRHEA

To soothe your bowels after an attack of diarrhea that has been sudden and quick to pass, herbal teas can be very helpful: try blackberry or peppermint tea for an astringent effect, fennel or marsh mallow for a soothing, healing effect.

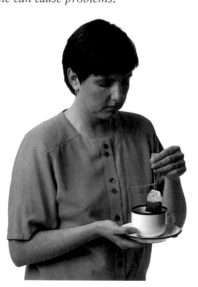

HERBAL TEAS
Warming herbal teas may prove beneficial for diarrhea. If you cannot find herbal tea bags, steep some fresh or dried herbs in boiling water.

Hot or warm drinks are better for inflamed bowels than cold ones; cold liquid passes very quickly through the body and can aggravate diarrhea. If you don't feel like eating, have warm, diluted apple juice or vegetable consommé instead. Diarrhea can easily dehydrate you, so drink plenty of fluids.

For diarrhea caused by an infection, eat yogurt with live cultures daily for a few weeks to restore friendly bacteria in the digestive system.

FOODS FOR CONSTIPATION

Constipation can be caused by insufficient dietary fiber or magnesium in the diet; poor fluid intake; a lack of exercise; or all four of the above. The solution is to eat more whole-grain breads, beans, vegetables, nuts, and brown rice—all fiber-rich foods that bulk up your stools. (They are also high in magnesium, which is important for proper bowel function, but can be offset by a high calcium intake.) The extra stool volume stimulates the muscles in the bowel wall to propel the contents along more rapidly. This process is known as peristalsis. The more rapidly the contents pass through the bowel, the less the bowel walls absorb fluid, and the softer the stools remain.

While extra fiber can help, too much all at once can irritate sensitive intestines and, in fact, have a constipating effect unless it absorbs plenty of fluid. It is essential to drink several large glasses of water every day.

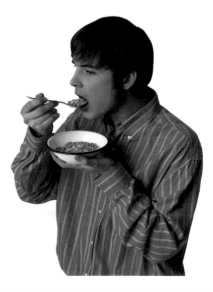

HIGH-FIBER CEREALS
Adding a bowl of whole-grain cereal to your daily diet can boost your intake of fiber and help stave off constipation.

REPRODUCTIVE AND URINARY SYSTEMS

Many problems of the urinary and sexual organs in both men and women can be improved through dietary management to restore the balance of health.

Imbalances in the body can lead to many types of problems, and the urinary and reproductive organs are not immune. Dietary deficiencies can increase a person's susceptibility to several disorders, even though these problems may not initially appear to be related to diet.

PAINFUL MENSTRUAL PERIODS (DYSMENORRHEA)

A number of women suffer abdominal cramps and bloatedness at the beginning of their menstrual period. Deficiencies of zinc, magnesium, and calcium all play a part in this susceptibility. Sometimes even mild deficiencies of these minerals, which may not show up in blood tests, can have an effect, so increasing these nutrients in the diet can help many sufferers.

Eating plenty of leafy green vegetables, nuts, seeds, legumes, and brown rice will ensure a better magnesium intake, while seafood will supply zinc. To increase calcium levels without increasing fat intake, eat low-fat or nonfat yogurt, calcium-enriched soy milk, and dark green vegetables.

Essential fatty acids, found in nuts and seeds, are necessary for the body's production of prostaglandin E_1, which encourages the muscle wall of the uterus to relax and relieves the pain of cramps. Evening primrose oil, available in capsules at health food stores, also contains an essential fatty acid and is sometimes recommended to relieve premenstrual and menstrual discomfort.

PREMENSTRUAL SYNDROME (PMS)

The hormonal changes that occur between ovulation and the start of menstruation are linked to fluctuations in blood sugar levels and changes in the levels of minerals and trace elements in the body. Many aspects of body function can be affected by these changes, giving rise to both emotional and physical symptoms of varying intensity.

Coffee, tea, colas, and alcoholic beverages can worsen anxiety symptoms and, in excessive amounts, may alter the balance of such hormones as estrogen. If you suffer from PMS, avoid these drinks for at least a week before your period is due. Although cravings can be strong just before menstruation begins, you should avoid sweets because they cause blood sugar levels to fluctuate rapidly (see page 146), making cravings worse and contributing to moodiness. To overcome cravings and relieve the associated *continued on page 114*

FOODS FOR ENERGY

Energy-rich foods can help you combat the worst premenstrual and menstrual problems by giving your blood sugar levels a steady lift and increasing your ability to confront your symptoms. High-fiber foods are advised for menstruating women (see page 113). An apple is a good source of fiber and some vitamins. A baked potato is high in complex carbohydrates and fiber, while a couple of plain rice cakes with peanut butter will boost fiber and protein levels.

APPLES
contain fructose, a simple sugar that is metabolized quickly, and pectin, which slows digestion and prevents a sudden rise in blood sugar.

POTATOES
supply potassium, essential for effective carbohydrate and protein metabolism.

PEANUT BUTTER
is a good source of niacin, important for energy production in the cells.

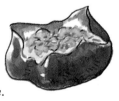

Premenstrual syndrome

The severity and duration of premenstrual symptoms can be lessened by cutting out certain foods during the week before your period is due and replacing them with alternatives that will actually improve your condition.

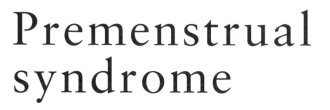

To prevent the discomfort of premenstrual syndrome, avoid foods that contain refined sugar. These cause blood sugar levels to rise rapidly and then drop just as quickly, thus contributing to the fatigue and moodiness of PMS. As well as the obvious sources, such as chocolate and cookies, watch out for hidden sources of sugar in breakfast cereals and other processed foods.

Caffeine can aggravate many of the symptoms of PMS, particularly headaches, anxiety, breast tenderness, and insomnia. To reduce the severity of these symptoms, limit your intake of tea and coffee to one or two cups a day and try alternatives, like herbal teas (raspberry leaf tea relieves cramps). If you are used to drinking a lot of strong coffee and decide to give it up, you may have withdrawal symptoms, such as mild headaches, for a day or two.

FRUIT RELIEF FROM PMS
Many women experience premenstrual syndrome with physical symptoms such as breast tenderness and excessive tiredness, as well as irritability, mood swings, and aggression. In the majority of cases, PMS can be treated successfully with diet, particularly vitamin-rich fruit snacks such as apples and pears. Diet changes should be tried before drug treatment is considered.

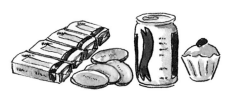

SUGARY FOODS
Low blood sugar levels, manifested as constant fatigue, can be exacerbated by sugary foods.

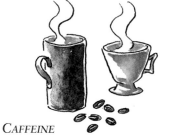

CAFFEINE
Headaches and insomnia, common premenstrual complaints, can be made worse by caffeine.

SPECIALIST ADVICE
If you suffer severely with PMS and do not experience any improvement after following the advice on this page, it could be that a food intolerance is making you ill. If you think this is the case, you will need special dietary advice. Ask your doctor to refer you to a registered dietitian.

SUPPLEMENTS FOR PREMENSTRUAL SYNDROME

Changing your diet is usually the most effective way of treating premenstrual syndrome, but occasionally women find that a particular supplement will help them. One widely used supplement found to be beneficial is evening primrose oil, which is available in pharmacies and health food stores. It is recommended particularly for relieving breast tenderness.

You can also ask your doctor or a naturopath to recommend a multivitamin supplement that is specially formulated for women who suffer from PMS. Vitamin B_6 is one important ingredient of such supplements. Remember that you should not take supplements for long periods of time without medical advice because some can be harmful in large doses.

Foods that are high in fiber

Increasing fiber in the diet can improve symptoms of premenstrual syndrome. Dietary fiber is a vital component of any healthy diet, but it is considered particularly important for women with PMS because it may help them excrete excesses of the hormone estrogen from their bodies. Blood estrogen levels are sometimes too high in women with PMS. A good intake of dietary fiber will not only help them lower it but also maintain their blood sugar at stable levels. This effect in turn can help stave off the exhaustion that many women experience prior to menstruation. The recommended daily intake of fiber is 20 to 35 grams, which can be obtained from having at least five to seven servings of fruits and vegetables, and at least two of whole-grain cereal products.

Foods that are high in minerals

Women with PMS should also eat foods that are rich in minerals, especially magnesium, iron, and zinc, because a deficiency in these can make PMS symptoms worse.

Foods that are rich in magnesium include all leafy green vegetables, whole-grain cereals and breads, brown rice, avocados, bananas, fish, and eggs. Nuts and legumes, such as peas, beans, and lentils, are also good sources of magnesium and can easily be included in your diet.

Foods that are good sources of both iron and zinc include red meats, such as beef, pork, lamb, and liver, also dried legumes, and shellfish.

Foods rich in essential oils

There are two polyunsaturated fatty acids—linoleic acid and linolenic acid—that are found in certain plants and are essential for good health. Furthermore, these oils have been found to help reduce premenstrual breast tenderness.

If you suffer from painful or tender breasts, on a regular basis try to include more leafy green vegetables, seeds (sunflower especially), and nuts in your diet and increase your use of such vegetable oils as corn, canola, safflower, or soybean for salad dressings and in cooking.

Eating regularly

During the week before menstruation begins, blood sugar levels can rise and fall dramatically. When they fall too low, a woman can experience dizziness, palpitations, sweating, and irritability. To maintain constant blood sugar levels and avoid these symptoms, try to eat something every three to four hours and choose fruit, bread, crackers, or cheese rather than a sugary snack.

RECIPES TO RELIEVE PREMENSTRUAL SYNDROME

Introducing the recommended foods into your diet may seem like hard work, particularly if you attempt it while you are suffering from the symptoms of PMS. Try instead to make gradual changes, incorporating one or two of the foods at a time or subtly altering favorite dishes to include the nutrients you need. The vegetable chili and the tuna and avocado salad below are simple and appealing ways to start you off.

VEGETABLE CHILI

2 tbsp vegetable oil
1 small onion, peeled and chopped
1 leek, sliced
1 clove garlic, chopped
½ green or red bell pepper, chopped
2 carrots, peeled and sliced
1 tsp chili powder
100 g /4 oz canned chopped tomatoes
100 g /4 oz cooked kidney beans
150 ml/²⁄₃ cup vegetable stock

■ Heat the oil in a medium saucepan over high heat; add the onion, leek, garlic, pepper, and carrots and sauté for 10 minutes. Stir in the chili powder, lower the heat, and cook 2 minutes more.
■ Add the tomatoes, kidney beans, and vegetable stock and bring to a boil. Cover and simmer for 30 minutes. Serve with brown rice.
Serves 2

TUNA, TOMATO, AND AVOCADO SALAD

1 avocado, peeled, pitted, and diced
170 g /6 oz water-packed tuna, drained and flaked
2 ripe tomatoes, diced
handful of lettuce leaves
½ red bell pepper, seeded and diced
1 hard-cooked egg, cut in wedges

For the dressing
3 tbsp sunflower oil
1 tbsp cider vinegar
freshly ground black pepper to taste
handful of chopped chives and parsley

■ Mix all salad ingredients except the egg in a large bowl. Prepare the dressing, pour over the salad, and toss well. Top with the egg wedges.
Serves 2

irritability or fatigue, eat yogurt regularly, consume fresh fruit between meals, and eat a light savory snack, like low-fat crackers, just before going to bed at night.

Supplements of magnesium, vitamin B_6 (as part of the B complex), and evening primrose oil have all proved beneficial in the management of PMS, in part because they help stabilize blood sugar levels and also because they increase the beneficial anti-inflammatory prostaglandin E_1, a hormone that helps to counteract some of the discomfort of the premenstrual phase.

TOFU BURGERS WITH TOMATO AND BASIL SAUCE

Soy products contain plant estrogens, which can help relieve menopausal symptoms. Fermented soy products, such as tempeh, miso, and tofu, are especially beneficial and are highly recommended ingredients for the menopausal diet.

For the burgers
1 tbsp sunflower oil
1 large carrot, peeled and finely grated
1 large onion, peeled and finely grated
1 clove garlic, crushed
1 tbsp tomato purée
225 g /8 oz soft tofu
25 g /1 oz fresh bread crumbs (1 slice)
25 g /1 oz (¼ cup) finely chopped nuts
freshly ground black pepper and salt to taste
sunflower oil for brushing

■ Heat the oil in a large skillet over high heat and stir-fry the carrot and onion for 3 to 4 minutes or until they are softened. Add the garlic and tomato purée and cook 2 minutes more, stirring constantly.
■ In a large bowl, mash the tofu with a potato masher and stir in the vegetables, bread crumbs, and nuts. Season with pepper and salt and beat until the mixture sticks together. With floured hands, shape into 8 patties.
■ Brush the patties lightly with sunflower oil and cook under a hot broiler for about 13 minutes on each side or until golden brown. Drain on paper towels. Serve immediately with the tomato and basil sauce and brown rice.
Serves 4

For the sauce
400 g /14 oz can chopped tomatoes
65 g /2½ oz (¼ cup) tomato paste
1 medium onion, peeled and finely chopped
1 clove garlic, crushed
1 tbsp dried basil, crumbled
freshly ground black pepper and salt to taste

■ Pour the tomatoes into a large saucepan and add the tomato paste, onion, garlic, and basil. Simmer, uncovered, for 20 to 30 minutes or until the sauce has thickened slightly and the onions are soft. Season with pepper and salt.
Makes about 750 ml (3 cups)

MENOPAUSE

When women reach menopause (on average around age 50), the ovaries dramatically reduce production of estrogen. This change can cause various symptoms, such as hot flashes, night sweats, and vaginal dryness. In the years following menopause, women become more vulnerable to heart attacks and osteoporosis (see page 46).

A combination of appropriate foods and plant medicines can help modulate the hormonal fluctuations and thus relieve symptoms and protect the body from other health problems at the same time. (You can consult a medical herbalist or naturopath for specific guidance in using herbs, a dietitian for nutritional advice.)

The severity of the symptoms experienced during and after menopause depend to some extent on genetic factors and overall health. A nutrient-rich, varied diet is the best way to sustain a healthy heart rate, good circulation, bone strength, and protection against the risk of cancer during this phase of life.

Important nutrients for preventing the ill effects of menopause are vitamins E and C, calcium, magnesium, and the essential fatty acids. (Caffeine and alcohol tend to deplete some of these nutrients, so intake should be minimized.) A few recent studies have suggested that some menopausal symptoms can be relieved by supplements of vitamin E. Evening primrose oil can also help relieve many menopausal symptoms, and similar relief can be found in such oils as canola and in pumpkin and sunflower seeds.

Substituting vegetarian proteins, such as beans and soy products, for meat and eggs will help you reduce your intake of saturated fat, which clogs arteries and increases the risk of heart disease and stroke. Soy products are also a very good source of natural estrogens, and foods rich in these can help to relieve or reduce the severity of menopausal symptoms. Statistics show that Japanese women living in Japan have a much lower incidence of breast cancer and menopausal disorders than those living in the United States. It is believed that this is because they eat more soy products and also oily fish, which are rich in omega-3 fatty acids, and consume less saturated fat.

CYSTITIS

The symptoms of cystitis, or inflammation of the urinary tract, include frequent urination with burning or irritation and cramps in the lower abdomen. Cystitis is most often caused by infection from the bacterium *E. coli,* which is normally present in the rectum and intestines and on the skin around the anus. The condition has also been associated with vaginal thrush (candidiasis) and occasionally food intolerance. It is aggravated by sexual intercourse. Cystitis may also be due to irritation or allergy caused by toiletries and soaps, spermicides, tampons, or a poorly fitting contraceptive diaphragm.

For acute cystitis the most important thing is to drink at least 2 quarts of fluids a day. Drink water as well as diluted apple, pear, or grape juice, unsweetened barley water, and parsley tea. Avoid all acidic drinks, including orange juice. Your diet should be alkaline and can include salads, steamed vegetables, or vegetable soup. For recurring cystitis, drink a glass of cranberry juice daily as a preventive measure.

Drinking a glass of water containing a spoonful of baking soda every day during an attack can make your urine alkaline and may prevent *E. coli* from multiplying. Avoid foods, such as meat and eggs, that create an acid climate. Do not drink coffee, tea, or alcohol until all symptoms are gone.

VAGINAL DISCHARGE

Around the time of ovulation, vaginal discharge naturally increases; an extra amount of discharge can also be an early sign of pregnancy. However, excessive discharge can signal an infection or unhealthy mucous membranes; if it is smelly or a strange color, you should seek an immediate consultation with your doctor.

Excessive vaginal mucus is viewed by naturopaths as a catarrhal condition affect-

CRANBERRY JUICE

Cranberry juice has become popular as a preventive measure for cystitis, although how it works is not fully understood. In 1994 Dr. Gerry Avorn and colleagues at the Harvard School of Medicine carried out a study of 153 older women who suffered from cystitis, to see if cranberry juice influenced the presence of bacteria in the urine. Those who drank 300 ml (1¼ cups) of cranberry juice every day for six months were 58 percent less likely to develop cystitis than those in a similar group who were given an identical-tasting placebo. The team concluded that cranberry juice can help prevent cystitis. Exactly why is not yet understood, but one theory is that it prevents

CRANBERRY RELIEF
A glass of pure cranberry juice can be a useful preventive treatment for cystitis.

bacteria from attaching themselves to the bladder walls, so that they are washed out in the urine. If infection has already set in, however, cranberry juice may mask the symptoms and allow the infection to worsen. Opinions differ, but some doctors believe it is better to drink it for preventing recurring infections rather than for treatment.

ing the mucous membranes in much the same way as nasal mucus does during a cold. Follow the suggestions on page 101 for reducing nasal mucus and increase your intake of foods rich in vitamins A and C, which will improve the health of the mucous membranes.

VAGINAL YEAST INFECTION

Vaginal yeast infection, also known as candidiasis and vaginal thrush, affects the mucous membranes of the vagina and is most often caused by an overgrowth of *Candida albicans*—a yeastlike fungus. The same fungus can also infect the mouth (the condition there is commonly termed "thrush") and the digestive tract.

Symptoms of vaginal yeast infection include a white discharge, often described as "cottage-cheese-like," and intense vaginal itching. Other symptoms may include diarrhea, bloating, flatulence, persistent headaches, the urge to urinate more often, skin rashes, and pain during intercourse. Diagnosis is usually made on the basis of symptoms alone because there are no reliable tests for the condition.

ESTROGEN
The female sex hormone estrogen (shown as a micrograph image, below) regulates menstrual changes in the body. It becomes depleted during menopause, leading to many of the characteristic menopausal symptoms.

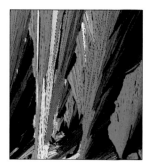

Candidiasis

Candidiasis, or vaginal thrush, is a yeast infection that can cause a number of unpleasant symptoms. A diet to beat it involves eliminating foods such as refined sugar and eating plenty of fresh vegetables and fruits that are low in sugar.

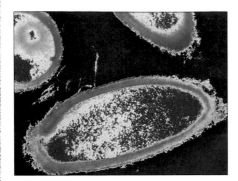

CANDIDA ALBICANS
This colored electron micrograph shows the bacteria found naturally in the gut and vagina that can cause candidiasis.

Candidiasis can, to some extent, be controlled by diet, but not all approaches are universally agreed upon. It is widely accepted that candida feeds on the simple carbohydrates in sugary foods. (Some naturopaths believe that it is also encouraged by fermented foods, like cheese and vinegar, and yeast-containing products, such as bread.) Treatment involves eliminating these foods from the diet. Once symptoms have disappeared, the problem foods can be gradually reintroduced.

If you suspect that you have candidiasis, you should seek advice from your doctor before embarking on any of the measures below.

PRACTICAL MEASURES

The following dietary measures can help relieve a yeast infection, as well as reduce the frequency of its occurrence. All except the very last item have been proved effective in various studies and are advocated by most health care professionals. If after following this diet for three weeks your symptoms have not improved, you should seek professional advice because you may have another type of infection.

- Cut out all types of refined sugars and foods containing them.
- Keep refined starches such as white flour to a minimum.
- Minimize fruits and fruit juices that are high in sugar, and increase your intake of those that are not, such as grapefruit (see below).
- Increase your intake of garlic; it contains an antifungal agent.
- Eat plenty of yogurt with live *Lactobacillus acidophilus* cultures.

These are friendly bacteria that can help prevent candida from getting out of control.
- Avoid drinks containing caffeine.
- Increase your intake of foods high in beta carotene, which boosts the immune system.
- Avoid foods that contain yeast and fermented foods that might contain it, such as beer, vinegar, and cheese.

FOODS YOU SHOULD EAT

The foods listed below contain important nutrients for good health. Increasing the amounts of these foods in your diet can help you avoid attacks of candidiasis.

Fresh fish and seafood; meat and poultry; vegetables and vegetable juices, especially carrots, cruciferous vegetables like cauliflower, broccoli, and cabbage, and leafy greens such as spinach; eggs; garlic; olive oil; linseed oil; millet; brown rice; wholegrain cereals; yogurt with live cultures; and legumes.

Cutting out fruit

Cutting out certain fruits and fruit juices will reduce your intake of important vitamins such as vitamin C and beta carotene. Because these cannot be stored in the body, you need to find alternatives that provide regular supplies. Eat more fresh leafy green vegetables, peppers, tomatoes, and watercress, aiming for at least five portions a day.

GRAPEFRUIT
Lower in sugar than other citrus fruits, grapefruit is less likely to encourage the growth of candida.

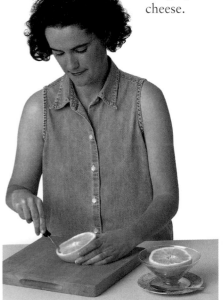

Many factors can alter the balance of microorganisms in the body, killing off the beneficial bacteria that normally maintain a healthy environment and encouraging candida. These include antibiotics, oral contraceptives, X-rays, poor digestion, chronic stress or illness, excess alcohol, a diet high in sugars and refined starches, steroid drugs, diabetes, douching, and hormonal changes during puberty, pregnancy, and menopause.

Candidiasis has been linked to poor diet in general, but especially to deficiencies of magnesium and zinc. Eating more foods that are high in these minerals—meat (especially liver), seafood, and dried legumes—will improve your immunity. So, too, will consuming foods rich in vitamins A and C, which are necessary for healthy mucous membranes, and the B vitamins.

Dietary management of candidiasis includes eating plenty of garlic for its antifungal properties and avoiding foods high in sugar because candida feeds on it. One head of garlic a day appears to be the most effective food; it should be chopped or mashed. To avoid sugar, it is necessary to read package labels carefully. The sugar in packaged foods may be listed as glucose, sucrose, fructose, maltose, dextrose, lactose, corn syrup, or molasses. Women who are severely affected by candidiases may even have to avoid fruits and fruit juices for a time.

Yogurt that contains live cultures, especially of the bacteria *Lactobacillus acidophilus*, has been shown in several studies to help prevent and promote recovery from yeast infection. The recommended amount is 1 cup per day.

BREAST-FEEDING

Breast milk is the finest nourishment for the human infant, containing all the elements a baby needs to thrive, develop, and stave off infection. To provide these benefits, breast-feeding should be continued for at least four to six months whenever possible.

FALAFEL WITH MINTED YOGURT SAUCE

Garlic and yogurt that contains live cultures are both known to help in the fight against fungal infections.

For the falafel
2 tbsp plain low-fat yogurt
  with live *L. acidophilus*
440 g/15½ oz can
  chickpeas, drained
100 g/4 oz fresh
  bread crumbs (4 slices)
1 medium onion, peeled
  and chopped
2 cloves garlic, crushed
2 tbsp chopped fresh
  parsley
freshly ground black
  pepper and salt to taste'
¼ tsp each ground cumin
  and coriander
2 tbsp flour
sunflower oil for frying

For the sauce
225 g/8 oz plain
  low-fat yogurt
4 tbsp chopped fresh mint
1 clove garlic, crushed
1 tbsp honey
freshly ground black
  pepper and salt to taste

■ Blend all the ingredients for the falafel except the flour and oil in a food processor or blender. Form the mixture into 12 small balls. Roll the balls in the flour and flatten slightly. Cover and let stand for 30 minutes.
■ Stir together all the sauce ingredients. Chill until needed.
■ Heat the oil and fry the falafel, a few at a time, for 2 minutes on each side; drain on paper towels. Serve hot with the sauce.
Serves 4

A less positive aspect of breast-feeding is that it draws heavily on the mother's nutritional reserves. For this reason it is important to follow a varied healthy diet during pregnancy and also during breast-feeding to prepare for and cope with the demands of breast-feeding. You can also prepare by increasing your intake of certain nutrients such as calcium. A balanced healthy diet should provide all the nutrition you need, but if you are unsure, ask your doctor or a dietitian about diet and about the possible use of supplements.

If your baby develops colic, diarrhea, or rashes, think about what you have been eating. Caffeine or alcohol should be avoided while you are breast-feeding, but certain foods can cause problems, too. For instance,

LACTOBACILLUS
The micrograph below shows Lactobacillis acidophilus *cultures taken from yogurt; these help to inhibit the growth of other bacteria that cause yeast infections.*

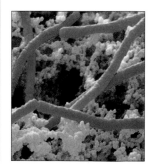

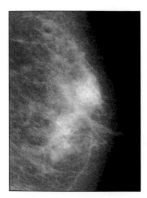

LUMPS IN THE BREAST
The majority of breast lumps, such as the one seen in the mammogram above as a white patch, are benign. This means that they will not develop into cancer. If you find a lump, however, you should see your doctor immediately for a diagnosis.

FOODS TO RELIEVE IMPOTENCE
Oily fish, nuts, seeds, and tahini are all excellent for boosting the production of testosterone, the male sex hormone.

wheat and cow's milk can, if not completely digested, stimulate the formation of antibodies that can pass through the breast milk and cause problems in the infant.

If you think that your diet may be affecting your baby's health, try excluding suspected foods, one by one, from your diet for a week or 10 days to see if your baby's problems clear up.

If any health problems persist or worsen suddenly during a period of self-treatment, either for yourself or your baby, seek professional medical advice as soon as possible.

BREAST PAIN

Pain or tenderness in the breasts can be caused by lumps or premenstrual swelling. In some women premenstrual breast pain is severe and may last for up to 10 days but should not be a cause for alarm. The majority of breast lumps are benign, but you should not hesitate to get the opinion of a qualified practitioner if you discover any new swellings in or near the breast.

Most forms of breast pain are thought to be associated with a sensitivity in breast tissue to the monthly fluctuation in female hormones. High levels of animal fats in the diet may exaggerate the effects of these hormones on breast tissue, and abstaining from foods such as meat and other sources of saturated fats may help relieve tenderness.

Some studies have shown that excluding coffee, tea, chocolate, and cola beverages from the diet alleviates the pain of breast lumps or premenstrual tenderness, but this is not effective for all women.

An adequate supply of essential fatty acids is known to reduce breast tenderness. These fats can be obtained from from sunflower and pumpkin seeds, flaxseeds, and polyunsaturated oils, such as canola and safflower.

IMPOTENCE

A man's inability to achieve or sustain an erection can be due to physical, emotional, or psychological problems. It may be a side effect of any number of disorders and is usually made worse by stress, anxiety, and fatigue. For cases in which impotence is the result of physical factors, dietary measures can bring significant improve-

ments. For efficient production of the male sex hormones, it is important to get certain nutrients in the diet including zinc, vitamin E, and the B vitamins. These nutrients are found in abundance in nuts, seeds, wheat germ, eggs, and whole grains such as millet, brown rice, and buckwheat. The benefits of these foods can be complemented with plenty of fresh vegetables and fruits.

Dates, seaweed products, yams, crabs, and lobster may also be beneficial because they too contain many nutrients that are essential to hormone production.

PROSTATE PROBLEMS

The prostate gland, which encircles the urethra in men, is found just below the bladder. Because of hormonal changes that take place with age, about 30 percent of men over age 45 develop an enlarged prostate, which can cause pain and urinary problems or may exhibit no symptoms at all. If trouble arises, it occurs usually at age 60 or later and is characterized by a need to urinate more frequently, accompanied by a sluggishness in starting the flow. As the prostate enlarges, it becomes stiffer and begins to cut off the flow of urine through the urethra.

Essential fatty acids have been found to relieve the discomfort of an enlarged prostate. Pumpkin and sunflower seeds and polyunsaturated vegetable oils, such as corn, safflower, canola, and linseed, are rich sources. Pumpkin seeds also contain zinc, necessary for a healthy prostate, and a substance called curcurbitacin, which is thought to curb the conversion of testosterone into dihydrotestosterone, which stimulates the prostate cells to proliferate.

Prostate cancer

Prostate cancer has been linked with a diet high in animal fat. To reduce the risk of developing prostate cancer, it is advisable to follow a diet low in saturated fats, the major type found in whole-milk dairy products eggs, and meats. This regimen will also help maintain a low-cholesterol level.

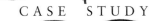

A Man with Prostatism

Problems with the prostate gland are generally noticed first when bladder control becomes erratic. The need to urinate with increasing frequency can be an inconvenience and a social embarrassment for older men. Fortunately, many cases can be helped by a combination of nutritional and herbal treatments.

Philip, now 68, has been enjoying retirement. It allows him more time to pursue his musical interest as a member of an amateur string quartet and to volunteer at a local hospital. All was going well until recently, when the need to urinate became more frequent and urgent, often waking him up several times during the night.

Philip has consulted his general practitioner, who has given him a careful rectal examination and a blood test. He was a bit tender on examination, and the doctor explained that this is caused by some enlargement and inflammation of the prostate gland, which is putting pressure on the urethra and bladder. Fortunately, the blood test ruled out prostate cancer.

WHAT PHILIP SHOULD DO

Philip's general practitioner, who has an interest in naturopathic medicine, has suggested that Philip try a dietary approach and herbal treatment to reduce inflammation and reduce his risk of developing prostate cancer. A dietitian will advise Philip on how to improve his eating habits, and an herbalist will recommend herbs that help reduce the prostate congestion.

He will need to cut down on sugar and alcohol and such stimulants as tea and coffee to reduce substances in the body that promote inflammation. Eating more foods high in esential fatty acids (vegetable oils and seeds) and zinc (seafood and sunflower seeds) will also help relieve his symptoms.

Action Plan

DIET
Substitute tofu, beans, and other vegetarian proteins for meat and eggs to reduce saturated fats.

HEALTH
Increase pelvic strength and circulation with regular brisk exercise. Follow the recommendation of the herbalist to take saw palmetto extract to help decrease frequency of urination.

EATING HABITS
Eat more foods that are rich in zinc and essential fatty acids, both of which help reduce symptoms of prostate enlargement. Also, cut back on animal fats.

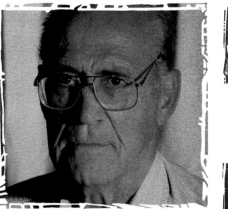

DIET
Many animal proteins contain a substance called arachidonic acid, which stimulates the formation of substances in the body that contribute to inflammation.

EATING HABITS
Swelling of the prostate gland can inhibit urination and increase nocturnal trips to the toilet.

HEALTH
The prostate gland is situated deep in the pelvic floor, where crowded organs and abdominal pressure can lead to sluggish circulation and poor drainage, plus swelling and inflammation.

HOW THINGS TURNED OUT FOR PHILIP

With time to prepare meals more thoughtfully, Philip adopted a diet that has helped to reduce his symptoms and lower his risk for developing prostate cancer. His herbalist's advice to take saw palmetto has also reduced swelling.

The need to urinate that had awakened Philip several times every night now happens, on average, only once a night, and a three-month checkup reveals that his prostate is a lot less tender and swollen.

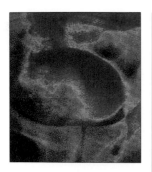

PROSTATE IMAGING
One way to get a clearer picture of prostate problems is with a special X-ray technique called intravenous pyelogram. The prostate shown above appears as a pale gold shadow against the dark red bladder, which has been injected with a radio-opaque liquid to make it easier to see.

Soy protein (in tofu and roasted soybeans) may protect the prostate from cancer. This is due to an estrogen-like substance in the plant that helps retard the growth of tumors.

Prostatitis

Inflammation of the prostate may come on suddenly, with a high fever and painful urination, or it may develop slowly and exhibit minor pain. Like any inflammatory condition, it will respond to a short cleansing diet—24 hours on vegetable and fruit juices, followed by two days of salads, steamed vegetables, and fresh fruit. As you return to a normal diet, incorporate into it plenty of foods rich in essential fatty acids; these help reduce prostaglandins, which cause inflammation. Also avoid spicy foods and alcohol.

INFERTILITY

Nutrition can play a small part in difficulties with conceiving. For example, food intolerances and deficiencies can be directly responsible for changes in mucus secretion in the vagina. Quite small changes in the vaginal acidity can make the environment hostile to a partner's sperm. Medical investigations are necessary to determine whether these or other circumstances are contributing to infertility.

Women who use oral contraceptive pills for a long time may suffer from vitamin and mineral deficiencies. In particular, a shortage of vitamin B_6 and manganese, both vital for the metabolism of estrogen, can lead to reduced fertility in women. Nuts, legumes, and all types of bran are good sources of manganese; foods rich in vitamin B_6 include green leafy vegetables, whole grains, potatoes, and meat, fish, and poultry.

Feeling run down or suffering severe stress may also impair the healthy function of sex organs. It is important to eat a healthy balanced diet and to seek nutritional advice if you suspect any deficiencies.

Recurring miscarriages have been linked to deficiencies of essential fatty acids, zinc, selenium, and vitamin E. Seek professional advice on improving your diet and do not take supplements without supervision.

Having a low sperm count or sperm that are too weak to fertilize an egg may be rectified by eating foods rich in zinc, as well as those that provide chromium, vitamin E, arginine (an amino acid), and essential fatty acids, all of which have been found to be low in people suffering from this disorder.

Foods rich in vitamin C, including citrus fruits, kiwifruits, currants, peppers, potatoes, and strawberries, may help prevent a condition known as agglutination, in which sperm become stuck together and are unable to reach the egg to fertilize it. This is a common cause of male infertility.

GENITAL HERPES

The type II herpes virus, which causes genital herpes, is closely related to type I, which is responsible for cold sores. Treatment with food is basically the same in both cases.

Foods high in vitamin C are essential to boost the immune system, and those with vitamin A to promote healthy mucous membranes. The amino acid lysine inhibits the virus and can prevent outbreaks or lessen their severity. Foods rich in lysine include fish, poultry, meat, especially pork, and cheese. Foods high in arginine (chocolate, nuts, and beer) seem to help the virus grow.

LEMON CHICKEN PASTA

Rich in lysine, chicken may help to inhibit the growth of the herpes virus, while the vitamin C from lemons boosts the immune system, which will help aid recovery from an attack.

1 tbsp sunflower oil
1 medium onion, peeled and chopped
4 boneless, skinless chicken breasts (115 g/4 oz each), cut into strips
juice of 2 lemons
175 g/6 oz low-fat ricotta cheese
100 g/4 oz mushrooms, sliced
350 g/12 oz pasta shells
chopped fresh tarragon

■ Heat the oil in a large skillet over medium heat; cook and stir the onion for about 5 minutes or until softened but not browned.
■ Add the chicken and cook for 3 minutes, stirring occasionally to avoid browning. Add the lemon juice and ricotta cheese and stir well until the mixture resembles a smooth sauce. Turn the heat to low, add the mushrooms, and cook, stirring occasionally, 6 minutes more.
■ Cook the pasta until al dente, drain, and turn into a warmed large serving dish. Stir in the chicken mixture and serve immediately. Sprinkle each serving with the tarragon.
Serves 4

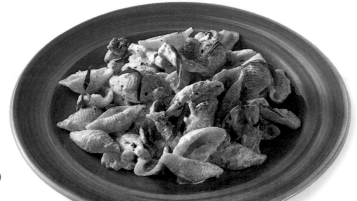

SKIN PROBLEMS

The skin is subject to both internal and external influences. Any reaction may have a multitude of causes, from dietary, bacterial, or hormonal changes to external factors, such as the sun.

A vital organ, the skin is dependent on nutrients from blood vessels and underlying tissue. In its contact with your immediate surroundings, the skin acts as a temperature regulator and protects all the organs that lie beneath it.

BRUISES

Bruising too easily may be the first sign of a deficiency of vitamins C and K, especially in the elderly. Broccoli, cabbage, and spinach are good sources of vitamin K and also vitamin C. Liver is an especially rich source of vitamin K. Some vitamin K is made by intestinal bacteria, which are promoted by lacto-fermented foods such as yogurt.

Older people can have a deficiency of stomach acid, which impairs absorption of some nutrients. Pineapple and papaya are good foods to promote better digestion.

SKIN CLEANSING FROM THE INSIDE

Many skin disorders respond well to a short cleansing diet. This one rests the digestive system and excludes foods that are likely to cause allergic reactions or food intolerance. When fruit juices are recommended, freshly squeezed ones are best, but unsweetened juices from concentrate will do.

If you have diabetes or any other metabolic disorder, seek medical advice before undertaking this regimen. This diet is not suitable for the elderly or children, and should not be followed more often than once every few months.

BURNS

There are degrees of severity in burns, but all burn victims should be given professional medical treatment and advice. The healing process makes extra demands on the body's nutritional reserves and reinforces the need for a diet rich in foods containing the antioxidant vitamins, A, C, and E, and the minerals sodium, potassium, calcium, and zinc to build up the immune system. Avocados, bananas, legumes, oranges, and vegetable stews are good sources of potassium, while calcium is plentiful in milk products, tofu, and leafy greens.

WHAT TO PUT ON A BURN

Always seek medical advice for serious burns because they are highly susceptible to infection.

▶ *Hold the affected part of the body under cool running water. Do not apply creams.*

▶ *For a mild burn, apply raw potato juice with a compress.*

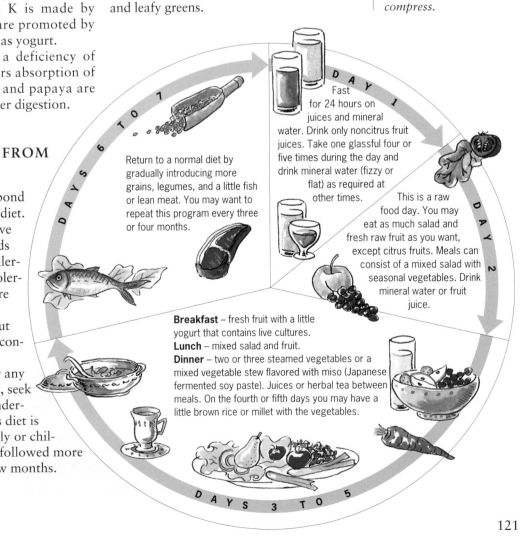

DAY 1 Fast for 24 hours on juices and mineral water. Drink only noncitrus fruit juices. Take one glassful four or five times during the day and drink mineral water (fizzy or flat) as required at other times.

DAY 2 This is a raw food day. You may eat as much salad and fresh raw fruit as you want, except citrus fruits. Meals can consist of a mixed salad with seasonal vegetables. Drink mineral water or fruit juice.

DAYS 3 TO 5
Breakfast – fresh fruit with a little yogurt that contains live cultures.
Lunch – mixed salad and fruit.
Dinner – two or three steamed vegetables or a mixed vegetable stew flavored with miso (Japanese fermented soy paste). Juices or herbal tea between meals. On the fourth or fifth days you may have a little brown rice or millet with the vegetables.

DAYS 6 TO 7 Return to a normal diet by gradually introducing more grains, legumes, and a little fish or lean meat. You may want to repeat this program every three or four months.

121

For anyone who has suffered extensive burns, a diet higher than usual in calories and protein from lean meat, poultry, sea-food, and eggs will help with tissue repair. Drinking plenty of fluids is also important. Diuretics such as coffee and tea should be avoided, as should alcohol, all of which leach fluids and important minerals from the body.

ACNE

Acne is an eruption of pimples, blackheads, and, occasionally, cysts that appear on the face, chest, and back. Hormonal changes are responsible for most cases of acne. For this reason it is primarily a disorder of youth, but it can occur in older people, too, especially in women, just before their periods, during pregnancy, or at menopause. Some medications can also cause acne. And stress can often trigger a flare-up.

Dermatologists stress that diet does not cause acne, but it can play a role in maintaining healthy skin. Of particular importance are vitamins C and A, which are also needed for efficient functioning of the immune system. Some studies have linked zinc to skin health. Zinc-rich foods include shellfish and meat.

A series of short cleansing diets (see page 121) in conjunction with a basic menu of abundant fresh fruit, vegetables, whole grains, and seeds, will provide the vitamins and essential fatty acids necessary for a healthy skin. An increase in vitamin E-rich foods, such as wheat germ and eggs, may help to heal skin that has erupted and reduce the chances of scarring.

Above all, eliminate from your diet any foods that seem to make your acne worse. Food intolerances and allergies can contribute to the problem.

ROSACEA

Rosacea, a disorder of facial skin that produces swelling, inflammation, and a chronic ruddy appearance, is not caused by diet but can be made worse by it. Spicy foods, especially, should be avoided, as well as alcohol, caffeine, and hot beverages, all of which have a vasodilating effect that can worsen the reddening.

Because rosacea patients have been found to produce less gastric acid and the digestive enzyme lipase, some nutritionists advise taking hydrochloric acid capsules and enzyme supplements. However, their effectiveness has not been proved.

Some rosacea patients are treated with longterm antibiotic therapy. It is recommended that they eat yogurt with live cultures or take acidophilus tablets to prevent an overgrowth of yeast.

ITCHING

Irritated, prickly skin is known as pruritis. It is sometimes a symptom of an illness, such as chicken pox, but in many instances itchy skin, with or without a visible rash, is caused by an allergy, a fungal infection, or chronic stress.

For many skin disorders, particularly those characterized by much irritation, excluding all foods that are high in sugar from the diet for two or three weeks may help to relieve itching. This includes soft drinks, malted beverages, wines, sherries, dried fruit, and canned foods with added sugar. A short cleansing diet (see page 121) may help improve the condition, start-

APPLE, APRICOT, AND CHEESE SALAD

Vitamins A and C may play roles in staving off the painful and often embarrassing signs of acne. This recipe contains these nutrients in a delicious combination.

2 firm eating apples
2 tbsp lemon juice
50 g/2 oz dried apricots, coarsely chopped
50 g/2 oz (2 medium stalks) celery, washed and diced
50 g/2 oz raisins
50 g/2 oz walnuts, roughly chopped
100 g/4 oz low-fat Edam or Gouda cheese, diced
¼ cup low-fat plain yogurt
¼ tsp cinnamon
few drops lemon juice
romaine or butter lettuce, shredded

▪ Wash, but do not peel the apples. Core, quarter, and cut the apples into bite-size cubes, put them in a large bowl, and toss them immediately with the lemon juice. Add the apricots, celery, raisins, walnuts, and cheese and mix well.

▪ Mix the yogurt with the cinnamon and lemon juice and stir it into the salad. Place some of the shredded lettuce on each of four salad plates and spoon the salad on top. *Serves 4*

ing with the 24-hour juice fast for adults and with day two, the raw food day, for children over the age of seven.

ECZEMA

Because eczema is often an allergic disorder, dietary approaches to it have been the subject of considerable investigation. Among the foods to which eczema sufferers are commonly allergic are cow's milk, eggs, and shellfish, while many cases are also aggravated by sugar and citrus fruits. Also, some food colorings, particularly the yellow and orange tartrazine colorings, can exacerbate eczema. Excluding these from the diet has proved beneficial in many cases.

A dramatic improvement may be achieved with a raw fruit and vegetable diet, which excludes possible allergy-causing substances and reduces the production of inflammatory substances in the body. Such a diet is not suitable for children.

It is also important to eat foods that provide adequate amounts of the nutrients that protect against inflammation and rashes. Zinc and the vitamin B complex assist the metabolism of essential fatty acids, which help prevent inflammation in the body. Intake of the essential fatty acids can be increased by eating nuts and seeds and cooking with sunflower, safflower, or canola oil.

Eczema often occurs with fungal infections, so you may benefit from increasing your intake of garlic and onions, which have antifungal properties.

PSORIASIS

Characterized by inflamed and thickened patches of skin, psoriasis is a common skin disease caused by new cells being produced far faster than normal and accumulating under dead skin patches. Although not an allergic disorder, psoriasis has been found to respond well to dietary changes.

Arachidonic acid, from meat products and dairy foods, is believed to promote the production of the prostaglandins that cause

LAMB KEBABS

Zinc and B vitamins, which are plentiful in lamb, may benefit eczema sufferers by helping to relieve inflammation. Here is a delicious and easy way to enjoy lamb for whatever reason.

5 tbsp lemon juice
5 tbsp soy sauce
1 clove garlic, crushed
450 g/1 lb lean lamb, cut into 4 cm/1½ in cubes
8 cherry tomatoes
12 button or small mushrooms, washed and trimmed
1 green bell pepper, seeded and cubed
8 pearl onions, peeled
half a small cabbage, grated
4 carrots, peeled and grated
2 small apples, cored (but not peeled) and diced
cooked brown rice

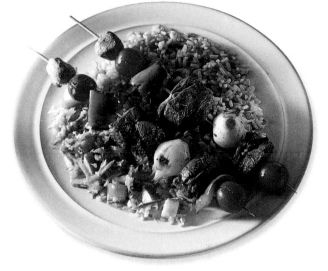

■ In a medium bowl, mix the lemon juice, soy sauce, and garlic. Add the lamb, cover, and marinate in the refrigerator for at least 2 hours.
■ Thread the lamb, tomatoes, mushrooms, bell pepper, and onions alternately onto long skewers. Cook the kebabs on a barbecue or under a hot broiler for 15 minutes, turning and basting with the remaining marinade until the meat is tender.
■ Boil any leftover marinade for 2 minutes and serve it with the kebabs. Serve on a bed of cabbage, carrot, apple, and brown rice.
Serves 4

the inflammation of the skin. Vitamin E, onions, and garlic are known to inhibit the uptake of arachidonic acid. Vitamin E is found in vegetable oils, nuts, and avocados.

Recent investigations into the effects of omega-3 fatty acids on psoriasis show a little promise. These fats, found in oily fish, seem to block the formation of prostaglandins, which play a role in inflammation. Exactly why omega-3 might improve psoriasis is not understood, but some patients have benefited from omega-3 supplements.

Many sufferers have difficulty producing vitamin D in their bodies and their psoriasis has improved after periods in the sun, which enables the body to produce vitamin D.

JOINT AND MUSCLE PROBLEMS

A main feature of joint and muscle problems is the pain caused by inflammation. This can be reduced by easing pressure on the affected area and following special dietary guidelines.

Iron loss

Many rheumatoid arthritis patients who take steroid drugs or painkillers like aspirin are prone to iron deficiency because of the medication. It is important for them to eat foods rich in iron and to have regular check-ups for anemia and related disorders.

Research shows that the food you eat plays a major role in the production of substances that promote inflammation in the body. Oily fish, which are rich in omega-3 fatty acids, are believed to reduce swelling, as are vitamin E-rich foods, such as wheat germ and nuts.

Excess pressure on the inflamed joints can exacerbate the problems. This pressure may be due to obesity, which causes the hips, knees, and ankles to carry an increased burden of weight. Repetitive movements, such as typing or playing a musical instrument, can worsen inflammation, and pressure from trying to force muscles to move as they should can add to muscle problems.

Allowing the affected muscles to remain unused, however, can cause them to waste away, or can lead to further problems as other muscles are used to compensate for those that are affected. Although dietary changes may bring relief from the pain of joint and muscle problems, always seek professional medical advice about long-term or worsening conditions.

ARTHRITIS

There are many types of arthritis but nearly all have been found to improve with dietary treatment of one sort or another. The two most common forms are osteoarthritis and rheumatoid arthritis, both of which are more common in women than in men.

Nutritional approaches to arthritis can be complex and individual requirements can vary enormously. It would be wise, therefore, to seek professional advice from a doctor who specializes in nutritional approaches or a naturopath if your symptoms worsen, you have any questions about treatment, or if the simple measures suggested here are not sufficiently effective

Avoid sugar

A first essential is to avoid sugar and refined flours. This is particularly important for anyone who is overweight. Excess weight

---

ARTHRITIS

Osteoarthritis is the medical name for the wear and tear of joints common in old age. The results of osteoarthritis are stiffness of the joints, difficulty and pain in moving, and sometimes deformity.

Rheumatoid arthritis is the term for an autoimmune disease in which the body's own immune system attacks the joints and the tissue around them, causing them to become inflamed and damaged.

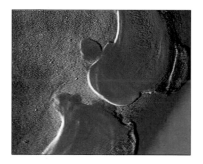

OSTEOARTHRITIS
The uneven edges where the bones meet show where the joint has been worn away.

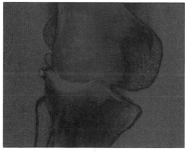

RHEUMATOID ARTHRITIS
The bulbous blue area to the right of the upper bone shows the area of swelling in the joint.

Pathway to health

A cabbage poultice can help to reduce the swelling of painful joints. Crush a few leaves of raw cabbage with a rolling pin or chop finely. Wrap in muslin to make a poultice and apply to painful or swollen joints overnight for several nights.

HOT OR COLD ARTHRITIS

In traditional Chinese medicine arthritis is classified according to the dominating symptoms. Foods to ease the condition are selected according to the Chinese belief in their properties of cooling or warming the body.

COLD-TYPE
Stiffness, worse on resting, dull aches worse in cold weather
Foods to eat: *garlic, onions, pepper, sesame seeds, lamb, ginger, spicy foods*
Foods to avoid: *cold foods, raw foods*

WIND-TYPE
Pains move about the body
Foods to eat: *grapes, black beans, whole grains, leafy green vegetables*
Foods to avoid: *meat, shellfish, sugar, alcohol*

DAMP-TYPE
Pain and swelling, inflammation, worse with movement
Foods to eat: *barley, mung beans, sprouted grains, millet, rice*
Foods to avoid: *cold foods, raw foods, dairy foods, meat, citrus fruit*

HOT-TYPE
Burning joints with little swelling, joints creak, stiff after rest
Foods to eat: *fresh fruits and vegetables, cabbage, sprouted soybeans*
Foods to avoid: *alcohol, spicy foods, onions*

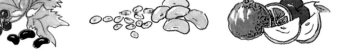

imposes an unnecessary burden on the ankles, knees, and hips. An excessive intake of sugar also affects the balance of calcium in the body, as do caffeine, tea, and bran. Replace caffeinated drinks with herbal teas or decaffeinated ones.

Food intolerance
Thought to be a significant factor in rheumatoid arthritis, food intolerance is believed to trigger the immune system, causing it to attack the joints. Commonly implicated foods in rheumatoid arthritis are wheat, oats, eggs, coffee, cow's milk, cheese, and meat, especially beef and pork.

This was emphasized by a series of Scandinavian studies, reported in 1991, which found that arthritis sufferers on vegetarian diets who also avoided wheat remained significantly better than control groups following a normal diet. In other research arthritis sufferers have improved on diets that exclude members of the nightshade family, such as tomatoes, eggplants, peppers, paprika, and potatoes.

Protective nutrients
At least two kinds of oil help fight inflammation: omega-3 fatty acids, found in coldwater fish, and gamma linolenic acid (GLA), derived from evening primrose, borage, and black currant seeds. Medical researchers have reported marked reduction in joint swelling, pain, and redness when rheumatoid arthritis patients take these oils. GLA can be taken in capsule form. However, doctors advise getting omega-3 from two or three servings of oily fish a week rather than supplements because excessive amounts of omega-3 can be hazardous.

Arthritis sufferers can also benefit from citrus and other fruits for their vitamin C content, which boosts the immune system, and also for their flavonoids, which may

SUMMER FRUIT COMPOTE

Berries are renowned for their rich flavonoid content. Some flavonoid compounds may relieve the swelling and pain associated with arthritis.

900 g/2 lb fresh summer fruits, such as cherries, blueberries, blackberries, and raspberries, or the equivalent weight in frozen, dry-pack fruits
1 tbsp arrowroot or cornstarch
apple juice or honey to sweeten (optional)
90 ml/6 tbsp low-fat plain yogurt

■ Place the fruits in a large saucepan and heat for 8 to 10 minutes, stirring occasionally, until the juices begin to run but the fruits still retain their shape.
■ Remove from the heat. Mix the arrowroot with a little water and stir into the fruit. Add apple juice or honey to sweeten if desired.
■ Cool before chilling thoroughly. Serve in glasses, topped with the yogurt.
Serves 4

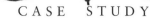
A Sportswoman

Nutritional deficiencies may become evident only after a long prelude of poor dietary habits, especially after exerting extra physical or mental demands on the body's resources. For men and women who engage in vigorous physical activity, it is particularly important to pay attention to eating well.

Annie is 38, unmarried, lives alone, and indulges her passion for sports. Because her work as a computer analyst is sedentary she likes to run three or four times a week. She has been rather concerned lately by attacks of cramps, which have stopped her in her tracks, once toward the end of a half-marathon and twice while playing squash.

Annie is in the habit of having fast-food lunches with colleagues, and in the evenings she usually warms up a small canned or frozen dish for a quick meal before she goes out for a run, believing that she needs it for energy. Having read a little about the role of nutrition she started taking a multi-mineral supplement but has not noticed much benefit.

WHAT SHOULD ANNIE DO?

The physical demands of Annie's sports activities are probably not being met adequately by her diet. She needs some professional advice on improving her eating habits.

A specialist in nutritional medicine could arrange tests to determine the levels of minerals and trace elements in her system. This would help determine if she actually needs supplements and, if so,which ones would be appropriate for her needs.

She needs to substitute fresh fruit, vegetables, low-fat dairy products, and whole-grain cereals for the fast foods, packaged convenience foods, and soft drinks that she typically relies on. She should also plan her meals more carefully in regard to her sports activities.

Action Plan

HEALTH
To improve digestion and replenish the nutrients vital for energy, drink pure juices and herbal teas instead of coffee, colas, and beer

DIET
Eat more fresh fruits, as well as vegetables with pasta, rice, or potatoes for healthier meals.

EATING HABITS
Plan to eat meals at least one hour after exercise. have a substantial lunch that includes protein and a healthful snack in the late afternoon to provide energy for running in the evening.

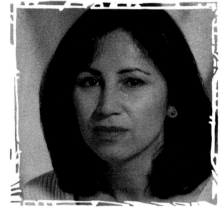

DIET
Many convenience foods are short of essential nutrients and are often high in fats and sugar.

HEALTH
Consumed regularly, alcoholic and sugary soft drinks will deplete the body of essential nutrients by replacing nutrient-rich calories with empty ones.

EATING HABITS
Doing physical exercise too soon after eating may contribute to cramping because blood needed by the muscles is still concentrated around the digestive organs.

HOW THINGS TURNED OUT FOR ANNIE

Once she got into the routine, Annie found that preparing a substanatial salad, pasta, or rice dish for lunch was not too difficult. She packed yogurt and fresh fruit for her afternoon snack and found these provided a better foundation for early evening training.

The tests had shown some deficiency of magnesium and zinc, so the doctor prescribed a suitable supplement to build up their levels, and cramps became a thing of the past.

SKELETAL MUSCLES

Cramps tend to affect the skeletal, or voluntary muscles, so called because they are under conscious control. Cramps can occur in muscles that are overused or tensed for long periods, or not receiving sufficient oxygen.

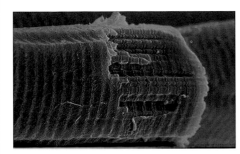

MUSCLE FIBERS
The muscles in the body are made up of fiber, like those of skeletal muscles pictured above. When these go into spasm, the effect is known as a muscle cramp.

have an anti-inflammatory effect. Ginger is also anti-inflammatory. Although more research still needs to be done, some studies indicate that beef, fatty foods, and vegetable oils high in omega-6 fatty acids can worsen arthritis inflammation in some patients.

BURSITIS

Inflammation of the muscle sheaths that lie near the joints is called bursitis, and it most commonly occurs in the shoulders, knees, and elbows. Bursitis can be caused by friction, pressure, or injury to the membrane around the joint.

Bursitis has responded favorably to intramuscular injections of vitamin B_{12}, and increasing the amount of vitamin B_{12} in your diet may also have a positive effect. Meats are rich in this vitamin; vegetarians can rely on soy milk enriched with B_{12}, fermented soy products, eggs, and dairy products. These foods, along with essential fatty acids and vitamin C to counteract inflammation, may help ease the pain of bursitis.

MUSCLE CRAMP

Most common in the legs, arms, and back, muscle cramps occur when the muscle fibers have insufficient oxygen, either from excessive exercise or when blood flow slows down, as for example, in bed at night. It is

also caused by an imbalance in the body of the minerals sodium, magnesium, calcium and potassium, rather than a lack of sodium alone, as is sometimes thought.

A diet based on vegetables and fruits that have lots of potassium and magnesium will help reduce the tendency to cramp, as will adequate vitamin E (found in vegetable oils, nuts, seeds, and avocados), which helps prevent oxygen deficiency in the muscles.

CANNELLONI IN TOMATO SAUCE

Vitamin B_{12}, plentiful in cheese, has been shown to ease bursitis. This recipe is an ideal source of B_{12} for lacto-vegetarians.

400 g/14 oz can chopped tomatoes
4 tbsp olive oil
2 cloves garlic, crushed
3 tbsp chopped fresh basil
1 bay leaf
freshly ground black pepper and salt to taste
12 dried cannelloni
100 g/4 oz (1 small) onion, peeled and finely chopped
175 g/6 oz minced protein substitute (textured soy protein)
140 g/5 oz (1¼ cups) freshly grated Parmesan cheese
1 tsp grated lemon rind
50 g/2 oz sun-dried tomatoes in oil, drained and chopped
25 g/1 oz toasted pine nuts, chopped
75 g/3 oz ricotta cheese
15 g/1 tbsp margarine
15 g/2 tbsp flour
300 ml/1¼ cups low-fat (1 percent) milk
basil leaves for garnish

■ Preheat the oven to 190°C/375°F. Place the tomatoes, half the oil, half the garlic, half the basil, the bay leaf, and the pepper and salt in a medium saucepan. Bring to a boil, then simmer, uncovered, for 30 minutes.

■ Meanwhile, bring a large pan of water to a boil, add the cannelloni, return to a boil, and cook for 10 to 12 minutes or until the pasta tubes are just cooked. Drain, refresh under cold water, and pat dry.

■ Heat the remaining oil in a skillet, add the onion and remaining garlic and sauté for 5 minutes. Add the soy protein and stir-fry for 3 to 4 minutes more. Stir in 2 tablespoons of the Parmesan, the lemon rind, tomatoes, pine nuts, the remaining basi, and the ricotta.

■ Place the margarine, flour, and milk in a small saucepan, bring to a boil, whisking constantly, then add ¼ cup of the Parmesan.

■ Stir 2 to 3 tablespoons of white sauce into the soy mixture and use it to fill the pasta.

■ Remove the bay leaf from the tomato sauce and divide the sauce among four ovenproof dishes. Place 3 stuffed cannelloni in each dish, pour the white sauce over, and sprinkle with the remaining 1 cup of Parmesan. Bake for 20 minutes or until bubbling and golden. Serve at once, garnished with basil leaves.

Serves 4

METABOLIC PROBLEMS

Some problems with the way the body processes and expends energy are partly the result of genetics and require medical attention; others can be prevented or relieved through diet.

With metabolic disorders, such as diabetes, hypoglycemia, and thyroid disease, the body's ability to regulate certain bodily functions is impaired. Dietary measures can often complement the medical treatment of these conditions.

DIABETES

A serious chronic disease, diabetes has two main forms: type I, which develops in childhood, and type II, which develops in middle age or later. With type I diabetes the pancreas fails to secrete sufficient insulin, the hormone that converts sugar to the energy required throughout the body. With type II there is no shortage of insulin but the tissues are insensitive to its action. All cases of diabetes require medical supervision because instability of the blood sugar levels can have serious long-term consequences. Diabetics are at greater risk for heart disease and kidney, eye, and neurological problems.

Many studies of diabetics have shown them to be deficient in hydrochloric acid (a substance secreted by the stomach that is essential for digestion) and, as a possible consequence of this, to have deficiencies of trace elements such as chromium, copper,

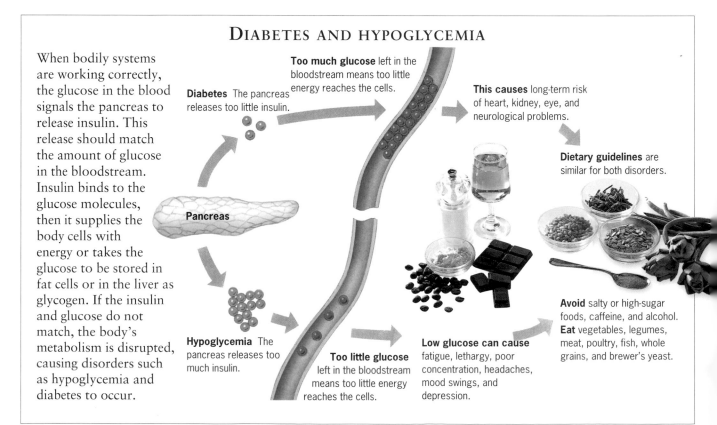

DIABETES AND HYPOGLYCEMIA

When bodily systems are working correctly, the glucose in the blood signals the pancreas to release insulin. This release should match the amount of glucose in the bloodstream. Insulin binds to the glucose molecules, then it supplies the body cells with energy or takes the glucose to be stored in fat cells or in the liver as glycogen. If the insulin and glucose do not match, the body's metabolism is disrupted, causing disorders such as hypoglycemia and diabetes to occur.

Diabetes The pancreas releases too little insulin.

Too much glucose left in the bloodstream means too little energy reaches the cells.

This causes long-term risk of heart, kidney, eye, and neurological problems.

Dietary guidelines are similar for both disorders.

Pancreas

Hypoglycemia The pancreas releases too much insulin.

Too little glucose left in the bloodstream means too little energy reaches the cells.

Low glucose can cause fatigue, lethargy, poor concentration, headaches, mood swings, and depression.

Avoid salty or high-sugar foods, caffeine, and alcohol. **Eat** vegetables, legumes, meat, poultry, fish, whole grains, and brewer's yeast.

CAUTION
For diabetics who are dependent on drugs or insulin injections, blood sugar levels can change rapidly. In order to keep the levels stable, such people need to eat regular carbohydrate-rich meals. Any dietary changes must be carefully monitored with regular checks of blood sugar levels. As fiber and complex carbohydrates or foods rich in chromium are increased in the diet, the need for insulin may be reduced, but medication should not be altered without medical supervision.

manganese, and zinc. Supplementing these nutrients in the diet has helped to improve the management of diabetes in many cases.

Diet control

Beyond the essential exclusion of sugar from the diet and the mandatory regularity of meals, careful attention to other aspects of dietary intake can often improve the degree of control over diabetes.

Research has shown that diets high in fiber and complex carbohydrates dramatically improve control of diabetes and may reduce the need for drugs in people who are suffering from type II.

All legumes, such as lentils, kidney beans, and peas, are especially beneficial because of their high fiber, high carbohydrate and moderate protein content. They can improve all aspects of diabetic control.

Chromium, which works with insulin to metabolize glucose in the blood, is found in brewer's yeast, liver, cheese, nuts, mushrooms, and whole grains, all of which are useful additions to the diet of the diabetic.

It is very important that people avoid becoming overweight if they have diabetes, or have a high risk of developing it because of a family history of the disorder. The sensitivity of the tissues to insulin is decreased in fatty tissue, so obese diabetics may need more insulin. Many overweight diabetics could reduce their insulin dependence by shedding some pounds.

If you are diabetic you should eat regular meals to maintain steady blood sugar levels and try to achieve a balanced diet that has limited sugar, fat, and alcohol. You should also keep salt and salty foods to a minimum because sufferers of diabetes are prone to

high blood pressure. Always read food labels carefully and be alert for any hidden salt and sugar in packaged foods.

Diabetic neuropathy

Diabetics are particularly susceptible to deterioration of the nervous system, especially in relation to the eyes and the nerves at the body's extremities. Poor eyesight and numbness of the hands and feet are common occurrences in older people with diabetes and may be overlooked as a sign of the onset of the disorder. If you have concerns about failing eyesight or circulation problems, see your doctor as soon as possible.

Some sufferers of diabetes have shown improvement in the nerves of the hands and feet with regular administration of evening primrose oil and vitamins of the B complex, especially thiamine (B_1) found in rice bran, millet, and brewer's yeast.

NUTTY LENTIL AND BULGUR SALAD

Lentils and bulgur can form an important part of a diabetic diet because of their high carbohydrate and fiber contents, which help regulate blood sugar levels and leave the body feeling satisfied.

150 g/5 oz bulgur
75 g/3 oz lentils
1 tbsp sunflower oil
1 medium onion, peeled and finely chopped
2 cloves garlic, crushed
4 medium tomatoes, roughly chopped
50 g/2 oz pine nuts
2 tbsp tomato sauce
1 tsp ground coriander
1 tsp ground cumin
2 tbsp chopped fresh parsley
2 tbsp lemon juice
freshly ground black pepper and salt to taste

■ Cover the bulgur with boiling water and soak for 30 minutes, then drain well. Meanwhile, cook the lentils in water for 30 to 40 minutes or until tender; drain well.

■ In a large skillet, heat the oil and sauté the onion and garlic for 4 to 5 minutes. Add the chopped tomatoes and pine nuts and cook 5 minutes more. Add the tomato sauce, lentils, and bulgur and mix well.

■ Stir in all remaining ingredients and heat the mixture through. Serve warm or chilled.
Serves 4

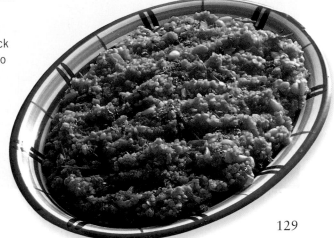

HYPOGLYCEMIA

Hypoglycemia is a disorder in which blood glucose levels fluctuate abnormally. The symptoms include hunger, fatigue, palpitations, poor concentration, headaches, weakness, dizziness, tremors, irritability, tension, confusion, and cold sweat. With so many symptoms that resemble those of other disorders, it is easy to misdiagnose this condition. Fortunately, many cases can be improved by dietary management.

MILLET AND AVOCADO BAKE

Thiamine (vitamin B₁) found in millet, is thought to help alleviate diabetes-related numbness in the hands and feet that sometimes occurs in older people suffering from the disease. This dish is a delicious way to increase your millet intake.

100 g/4 oz millet
4 ripe avocados
3 tbsp lemon juice
150 g/5 oz plain low-fat
  yogurt
50 g/2 oz (1/2 small)
  onion, roughly
  chopped
2 egg yolks
1 egg white
25 g/1 oz fresh
  bread crumbs (1 slice)
¼ tsp ground paprika
freshly ground black
  pepper and salt to
  taste
2 or 3 oranges

■ Preheat the oven to 200°C/400°F. Add the millet to a large pan of boiling water. Lower the heat, cover, and simmer for 30 minutes or until tender. Drain well.
■ Cut the avocados in half and remove the pits. Carefully scoop the flesh out of three avocado halves with a large spoon, leaving a thin layer of flesh in the shells. Slice the flesh thinly and reserve the shells. Toss the avocado slices with two 2 teaspoons of the lemon juice. Cover tightly and refrigerate.
■ Scoop out the remaining avocado flesh as before and reserve the shells. Put the cooked millet, avocado flesh, remaining lemon juice, the yogurt, onion, and egg yolks in a food processor and blend until smooth. Turn the mixture out into a bowl. Stir in the bread crumbs, paprika, pepper, and salt.
■ Whisk the egg white until stiff but not dry and fold into the avocado mixture. Divide the mixture among the 8 avocado shells and arrange them in a shallow ovenproof dish.
■ Bake for about 35 minutes or until puffed and golden. Serve with orange segments and the reserved avocado slices.

Serves 4

By contrast with diabetes, which is caused by too little insulin, hypoglycemia is the result of excessive insulin secretion, often from a pancreas that has been sensitized by dietary abuse, such as excessive sugar, alcohol, or caffeine intake, over a number of years. Other factors, for example, a genetic tendency and prolonged stress, can also contribute to excess insulin production. The consequent lowering of blood sugar levels by the insulin starves the brain of energy and leads to mental and emotional symptoms as well as many physical effects.

Refined sugars, which are absorbed rapidly in the body, and stimulants like caffeine, may induce excessive insulin output, but some healthy foods with a high glycemic index (see opposite page) can trigger the same response in sensitive individuals. A diabetic can suffer a hypoglycemic attack when insulin dosage doesn't match sugar intake. In such a case, sipping fruit juice or sucking on a hard candy is a quick antidote.

Prolonged exposure to stress also compounds the problem by increasing adrenaline output. Adrenal hormones stimulate insulin secretion and contribute to the headaches, palpitations, and other symptoms that hypoglycemics experience.

There are several types of hypoglycemia. For accurate diagnosis and appropriate treatment you should consult a doctor or naturopath who can arrange for necessary tests. Dietary management can be tailored to your individual needs.

Dietary guidelines

The main objectives of dietary treatment for hypoglycemia are to reduce the amount of insulin produced by the pancreas and to provide sufficient slow-releasing sources of energy to sustain adequate blood sugar levels. It may also be necessary to increase the dietary intake of nutrients such as chromium and magnesium, which help to regulate glucose metabolism.

To sustain healthy blood sugar levels, eat meals high in protein and complex carbohydrates If you become irritable a couple of hours after eating, eat a small protein or carbohydrate snack mid-morning, mid-afternoon and before going to bed at night, so that blood sugar levels do not drop too low.

Avoid sugar and any foods that contain it. Also avoid stimulants such as tea, coffee, alcohol, and nicotine, because these can cause glucose levels to fluctuate. A study reported in 1993 found that people with hypoglycemic tendencies who consume caffeine can develop symptoms of hypoglycemia even when blood sugar levels are in the low normal range. Excessive alcohol consumption has the same effect. Caffeine and alcohol stimulate adrenal hormones, which exaggerate many symptoms of low blood sugar.

It is important to obtain professional advice on managing blood sugar problems and on the appropriate use of supplements such as magnesium, zinc, chromium, vitamin B complex, and vitamin C.

The Glycemic Index

Many common foods have been classified according to the degree to which they stimulate the pancreas to release insulin and the subsequent effect on blood sugar levels. The scale is based on the speed with which food is absorbed. Using glucose as the standard at 100, other foods are scored against it. Surprisingly, parsnips and carrots both score higher than honey, and some types of chocolate score less than a potato. At the lowest end of the scale are beans and soy products. People with hypoglycemia or diabetes should choose foods at the lower end of the scale. Thus, while parsnips, carrots, and whole-grain bread are healthy foods in normal circumstances, they have a high glycemic index and should be rationed, while fruit (containing fructose) is low and is acceptable in moderation.

THYROID PROBLEMS

The thyroid gland produces two important hormones that influence almost every function of the body. To create these hormones it needs iodine; too much or too little can cause the gland to malfunction. (Thyroid problems can also result from an hereditary disposition to them or an infection, tumor, or autoimmune disorder.)

A person with an underactive thyroid may exhibit unexplained weight gain, lethargy, muscle weakness, and memory problems. Someone with an overactive thyroid also experiences muscle weakness, plus weight loss, unusual hunger, and rapid hearbeat.

Iodine is found in seafood, dairy products, vegetables grown in coastal farmlands, and table salt that is enriched with it. Because of iodized salt, people in the United States rarely lack sufficient iodine.

TZATZIKI

This high-protein dip is a good choice for people who must regulate their blood sugar level. It can also be used as a sauce for baked potatoes or steamed vegetables.

150 g/5 oz cucumber (1 medium), diced
150 g/5 oz plain low-fat yogurt
8 to 12 fresh mint leaves
2 cloves garlic, crushed
freshly ground black pepper to taste

To serve:
fresh vegetables, cut into sticks for dipping

■ Mix the cucumber and yogurt together. Roughly tear the mint leaves and add them to the yogurt along with the garlic and pepper. Mix well and chill for at least 2 hours.
■ Serve with sticks of raw vegetables, such as bell peppers, celery, and carrots, or high-fiber, low-sugar crackers (see below).
Serves 4

OAT, WALNUT, AND SESAME CRACKERS

Low in sugar and high in fiber, these crispy crackers make a perfect snack. Serve them with tzatziki (see above) or eat them as they are, fresh from the oven.

150 g/6 oz whole-wheat flour
50 g/2 oz quick-cooking oatmeal
25 g/1 oz (¼ cup) finely chopped walnuts
25 g/1 oz sesame seeds
pinch of salt
75 g/3 oz corn oil margarine
1 to 2 tbsp low-fat (1 percent) milk

■ Preheat oven to 190°C/375°F. Put the flour, oatmeal, walnuts, sesame seeds, and salt in a large mixing bowl and rub in the margarine until the mixture resembles fine bread crumbs.
■ Add the milk, a little at a time, until the mixture forms a firm dough. Turn out onto a floured surface and roll out to ⅛ in thick. Use a 7.5-cm/3-in fluted cutter to cut into 16 rounds.
■ Place on a baking sheet and bake for 12 to 15 minutes, then transfer immediately to a cooling rack. Serve with cheese or a dip such as hummus.
Makes 16 biscuits

EMOTIONAL PROBLEMS

Many studies have shown that the resilience of the brain and nervous system is particularly affected by nutritional deficiencies, but dietary changes may help relieve symptoms.

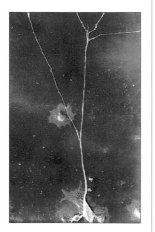

NEURON
The brain houses billions of neurons, which conduct electricity between cells.

The well-nourished mind is far more capable of acting rationally and calmly in most situations than one that is malnourished. The ability to make informed decisions, to be socially active, and to exercise control over impulses toward anger or aggression appear to be strongly influenced by biochemical factors that can be modulated by food.

ANXIETY AND TENSION

Stress is something your body is equipped to handle, but when it is prolonged, it can lead to a breakdown of various coping mechanisms and result in chronic tension or states of anxiety. When this happens you become vulnerable to other disorders, especially headaches, fatigue, skin complaints, musculoskeletal problems, and depression of the immune system, which in turn leaves you vulnerable to infection.

Many studies have shown that the resilience of the brain and nervous system is affected by nuritional deficiencies. There are various steps you can take if you feel that you are not coping as well as you could.

To help lower your anxiety threshold, cut back on coffee, strong tea, and cola drinks because excessive caffeine can result in jitteriness and erratic swings in blood sugar and mood. Caffeine leaches vital minerals from the body as well. Also, don't skip meals. If a hectic work schedule interferes with mealtimes, keep a stock of healthful snacks on hand—fresh fruit, low-fat yogurt, cheese, and whole-grain crackers, for example.

BRAIN ACTIVITY AND EMOTIONAL HEALTH

People suffering with emotional problems often have reduced levels of activity and blood flow in the brain, which can affect neuron transmission and lead to loss of concentration and sadness. Treatment can help improve brain activity.

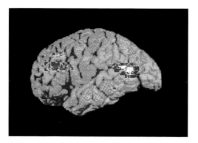

DEPRESSED BRAIN
The red and yellow areas in this brain indicate those regions where brain activity is at a particularly low level.

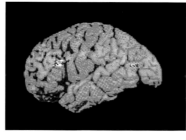

HEALTHY BRAIN
The brain pictured above shows that the areas of low brain activity are much smaller following treatment for depression.

Pathway to health

Coping effectively with stress is a skill that can be cultivated, and there are a number of ways of learning to let go of tension. With regular instruction and daily practice, it is possible to lower blood pressure and release more energy for constructive purposes.

Yoga, T'ai Chi, and Qigong are Eastern exercise systems that have all proved their worth in stress management. Other relaxation systems, such as autogenic training, can also be helpful in conatrolling stress.

Improving the quality and quantity of sleep is essential to reduce the toll of stress on your mind and body. Homeopathic remedy Arnica 6c may also help (see page 152) achieve this.

Stress

Stress is a common result of today's hectic pace of life—racing to meet a deadline at work, getting stuck in traffic, or rushing to complete the household chores. Such day-to-day stressors can build up and cause any number of stress-related disorders.

When extra demands are made on your energy, your body has to pump out stress hormones like adrenaline and cortisone to help you meet them.

Being stressed may mean you do not eat properly. At the same time, stress reduces the efficiency of your immune system, making a good diet even more essential.

The very foods that you turn to for convenience when time is short may be lacking in the nutrients that you need to cope with stress. For instance B vitamins, magnesium, and zinc are especially important for muscle

relaxation; if you do not get enough you can easily feel more on edge and less able to relax and sleep. In turn, this adds to the feeling of stress and creates a vicious circle. You need to eat wholesome foods: whole-grain bread, brown rice, vegetables, beans, and nuts, which are rich in the nutrients your body craves when stressed.

Heallthful foods do require a bit of planning, such as buying in advance instead of when you are hungry. When making a spur-of-the-moment decision you may be more likely to buy something like chocolate.

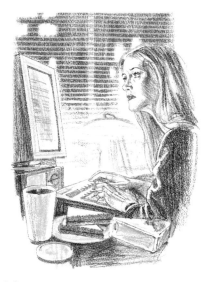

MEALS AT WORK
Not tearing yourself away from your desk to eat can leave you low on energy, limited in the ability to concentrate, and vulnerable to digestive disorders.

TIME-SAVING TIPS

If you restock your kitchen every week with wholesome foods that can be cooked or warmed up quickly, you are conveniently ready for good health. Brown rice or beans can be cooked in advance, stored in serving sizes in the refrigerator or freezer until needed, and reheated when you get home from work. Chicken and fish, frozen in individual portions, can be thawed in a microwave and cooked for dinner in a few minutes. If you do not even have time to peel vegetables, buy frozen. They can be

cooked in the same time it takes you to go buy a bag of chips and are a lot better for you. If you are short of ideas, there are lots of cookbooks that specialize in time-saving recipes.

In the evening prepare a healthful lunch to take with you the next day; you can wrap sandwich ingredients separately and put them together just before eating to prevent sogginess. Leftovers from dinner are convenient, especially made into a salad. Once you have a routine, eating healthfully will be easy and rewarding.

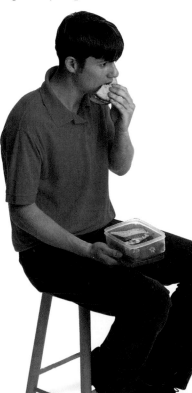

TAKING TIME
At school or the office it is important to make time to eat properly. This may involve preparing food the previous evening in order to enjoy a healthful and relaxed lunch.

TEN-MINUTE MEAL
With a little advance preparation, it's possible even with the busiest schedule to make a quick and healthy meal, such as grilled sole on a bed of brown rice, lentils, onions, and tomatoes.

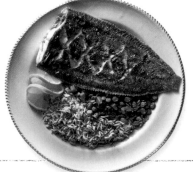

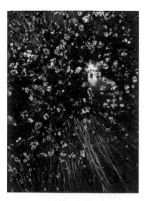

SEROTONIN
The chemical serotonin, shown above, is produced by the brain to assist in the transmission of messages from the nerves. It also helps lift mood.

The lactate connection

According to a report in the *International Clinical Nutrition Review*, 1985, lactic acid, usually produced by muscles as they are being worked vigorously, may be a major cause of panic attacks—extreme, short but intense bursts of anxiety. Some studies found that patients who were prone to panic attacks had blood lactate levels that were twice as high as those of control subjects, when tested after physical exercise.

Alcohol, caffeine, and refined sugar all increase lactate levels, while magnesium helps to reduce them.

Magnesium, potassium, calcium, B vitamins, and lecithin are nutrients that are essential to sustaining resilient nerves. You can obtain them from whole grains (millet, brown rice, whole-wheat bread), eggs, root vegetables, and soy products.

PASTA WITH TUNA–TOMATO SAUCE

High in tryptophan, essential for healthy serotonin production, and a good source of complex carbohydrates, this delicious meal may help beat the blues.

250 g/12oz pasta twists
1 tbsp sunflower oil
100 g/4 oz (1 small) onion, peeled and minced
1 clove garlic, crushed
450 ml/2 cups tomato purée
1 tbsp tomato paste
freshly ground black pepper and salt to taste
1½ tsp dried oregano
170 g/6 oz can tuna in water, drained and flaked
12 black olives, pitted and halved
50 g/2 oz sharp Cheddar cheese, grated (½ cup)
25 g/1 oz fresh bread-crumbs (1 slice)

■ Cook the pasta in boiling salted water and drain well; transfer to a flameproof casserole.
■ Meanwhile, heat the oil in a large nonstick skillet and sauté the onion and garlic for 4 to 5 minutes, stirring occasionally. Add the tomato purée, tomato paste, pepper, salt, and oregano to the skillet and mix well.
■ Preheat the broiler. Stir the tuna and olives into the tomato sauce and cook 5 minutes more. Pour the sauce over the pasta and mix well. Sprinkle with the grated cheese and bread crumbs. Broil until golden brown and bubbling.
Serves 4

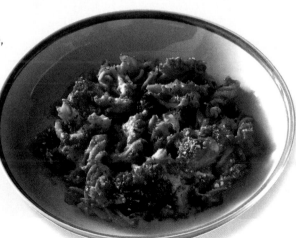

DEPRESSION

Depression can accompany physical ailments such as anemia, hypoglycemia (see page 130), an underactive thyroid gland, and intestinal candidiasis (see page 115), so professional help should be obtained if a depression persists for more than a week or two without apparent reason.

A biochemical basis has been suggested for some types of depression. The chemicals that transmit the electrical messages between nerve endings depend on a number of nutrients. Without these, the impulses are not transmitted as efficiently. Nutrients believed to be important include vitamin C, vitamins of the B complex, lecithin, calcium, magnesium, and potassium—all of which are obtained from a well-balanced diet.

The amino acid tryptophan must be present for the brain to form serotonin, a "feel good" chemical that participates in the transmission of nerve impulses. Tryptophan is found in a number of foods, especially in nuts, eggs, fish, turkey, and dairy products, but high-protein meals may block its availability to the brain because of competition from other amino acids. For this reason meals high in carbohydrates are considered more conducive to serotonin production, but the carbohydrates must be from slow-release sources like pasta and rice. These will also provide B vitamins, which promote healthy lactic acid bacteria in the intestines.

INSOMNIA

Difficulty in sleeping has been linked to fluctuations in blood sugar levels, other biochemical changes, and deficiencies of magnesium, copper, iron, and the B vitamins, especially niacin. Caffeinated drinks can exacerbate the problem. Because caffeine can take up to eight hours to be eliminated from the body, even a late-afternoon cup of coffee can keep a person awake at night.

A natural sleep inducer is tryptophan (see above). Tryptophan increases the amount of serotonin—a sedative—released by the brain. Since carbohydrates facilitate the entry of tryptophan into the brain, combining turkey with bread, cheese with crackers, or milk with honey, for example, will increase the effectiveness of the tryptophan.

Melatonin has been touted as a sleep aid. The taking of supplements is still controversial, but many foods, including bananas, rice, and corn, contain small amounts of it.

CHAPTER 6

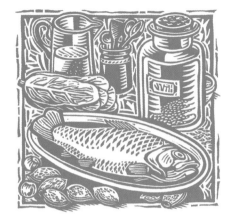

PLANS FOR HEALTH

Many illnesses, health conditions, and food intolerances can be successfully managed by adjusting the diet. Eating more of the foods that confer a specific nutritional benefit can improve symptoms significantly. Similarly, avoiding certain foods that cause or contribute to illness will relieve many conditions. Finding suitable substitutes for eliminated foods is a key to maintaining a balanced diet.

Blood-Pressure-Lowering Plan

Poor diet and being overweight are two of the many factors that contribute to hypertension. A diet aimed at lowering blood pressure focuses mainly on reducing sodium intake and increasing intakes of potassium and magnesium.

The main causes of high blood pressure are a combination of family predisposition and such factors as being overweight, having a poor diet and too little exercise, and drinking to much alcohol.

High blood pressure is often accompanied by atherosclerosis, a narrowing of the arteries that restricts the flow of blood to vital organs. This arterial narrowing can become worse if there is a buildup of cholesterol due to a high-fat diet. If high blood pressure continues untreated over a period of time, the risk of blood clots (thrombosis) forming in the narrowed sections of arteries increases. A clot lodged in a coronary artery may cause a heart attack, one near the brain, a stroke.

YOUR BLOOD PRESSURE
In a healthy young adult a normal blood pressure is around 120/80 mm Hg (blood pressure is recorded in millimeters of mercury, or Hg). The higher (systolic) figure refers to the blood pressure as the heart pumps out blood; the lower (diastolic) figure to the blood pressure between pumps. The upper limit of an acceptable blood pressure is 140/90. A blood pressure above this could present serious health problems.

LOWERING THE PRESSURE
Reducing your fat intake, cutting down on alcohol, and increasing physical activity can help to reduce your weight and bring your blood pressure down. It is also important to cut down on sodium intake. You can replace salt in dishes with herbs and spices to maintain flavor.

HOW MUCH SALT?
A certain amount of sodium is necessary for helping to control fluid balance, transmit nerve impulses, and contract the muscles. Eating too much now and then is not usually a problem: any short-term excess salt is dealt with by the kidneys, which simply excrete what is not needed. Problems arise, however, when you eat too much sodium on a regular basis. The actual need for salt is 200 to 300 milligrams a day, or no more than 1/8 teaspoon, but experts advise that between 2,200 and 3,300 (1 to 2 teaspoons) is still acceptable for most people. For the minority who are salt sensitive, this amount is too much.

THE MINERALS FACTOR
Potassium, calcium, and magnesium are minerals that play an important role in controlling blood pressure. Studies show that cutting sodium intake and increasing potassium and magnesium intake simultaneously can be more beneficial than simply the sodium.

REDUCING STRESS
Relaxation exercises can help keep your blood pressure levels stable. Breathing exercises and visualization techniques—focusing your mind's eye on a pleasant scene while you relax—can definitely help, but relaxing pastimes, such as painting or tending an herb garden, are also useful. An herb garden is doubly useful because you can use the herbs to flavor food as you cook it, instead of adding a lot of salt.

THE POSSIBLE EFFECTS OF HYPERTENSION

Hypertension, or high blood pressure, contributes to a number of disorders around the body. If left untreated, hypertension can increase the risk of circulatory problems and heart and kidney damage.

It is particularly important for pregnant women to watch their blood pressure. High blood pressure during pregnancy, called pre-eclampsia, can lead to the serious condition eclampsia, in which convulsions occur that can cause damage to the baby and coma and death for the mother.

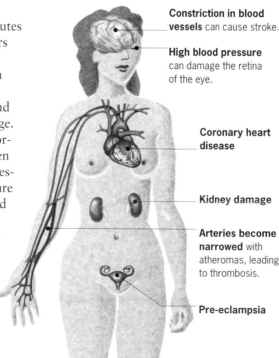

Constriction in blood vessels can cause stroke.

High blood pressure can damage the retina of the eye.

Coronary heart disease

Kidney damage

Arteries become narrowed with atheromas, leading to thrombosis.

Pre-eclampsia

STEP-BY-STEP RELIEF FROM HIGH BLOOD PRESSURE

1 *REDUCE YOUR SODIUM INTAKE.*
Cut down on high-sodium processed foods, such as breakfast cereals, dried and canned soups, and processed meat products. Get into the habit of checking food labels and replace salt in cooking with herbs and spices.

SALT ALTERNATIVES
Herbs are a flavorful, low-sodium alternative to salt in cooking. They can enhance your food without raising your blood pressure. A small herb garden is doubly useful because it requires little space, and tending the plants can be very relaxing and help to reduce stress.

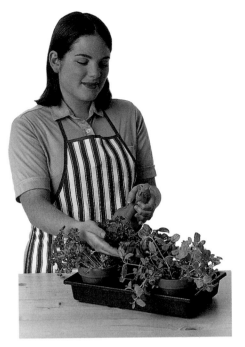

2 *EAT MORE MINERAL-RICH FOOD.*
Increase potassium in your diet with bananas, oranges, cabbage, broccoli, and peppers. Broccoli and milk products are good for calcium and whole-grain cereals, beans, and fruit for magnesium. (Note: milk is also high in sodium.)

3 *LIMIT YOUR ALCOHOL INTAKE.*
One or two drinks per day may help reduce your cholesterol levels, in turn bringing your blood pressure down. However, more than this can actually raise blood pressure over time.

4 *TAKE TIME OUT TO REDUCE STRESS.*
Manage your schedule better to make time for regular exercise. Moderate exercise, such as walking or cycling for 30 minutes three days a week, can help reduce stress and lower blood pressure.

Menu Ideas

Look for foods that have a low-salt content and try salt-free alternatives. If you use a lot of salt in cooking, try brands that contain a blend of potassium chloride and sodium chloride.

Breakfast
Choose an unsalted breakfast cereal that is rich in magnesium, such as wheat biscuits. Low-fat yogurt with fresh fruit and oatmeal with dried fruit offer healthy alternatives.

Lunch
Have a baked potato with a topping of chili and combine it with a salad made with a low-fat yogurt dressing. Or prepare homemade vegetable or lentil soup with salt-free vegetable-stock concentrate.

Dinner
Cut down on frozen, packaged, and take-out meals because these tend to be very high in salt. Prepare your own meat, fish, pasta, and vegetable dishes, flavoring them with onions and garlic, basil and other herbs, coriander and other spices. Salsa is especially good for replacing salt.

MIXED SALAD WITH RICE
Cut your consumption of saturated fats with a refreshing mixed salad that is rich in minerals like potassium. Choose a low-salt salad dressing or mix your own with lime or lemon juice, oil, and tabasco sauce.

Peppers are a rich source of potassium, beneficial in controlling your blood pressure.

Herbs add delicious flavor to salads without increasing the sodium content.

Snacks
Choose crackers, nuts, popcorn, or rice cakes labeled low-salt or no salt. Low-fat yogurt mixed with dried or fresh fruit makes a delicious calcium-rich snack. Fresh fruit is always a winner.

Rice is naturally low in sodium and contains potassium and some magnesium, which can help to control blood pressure.

Cholesterol-Lowering Plan

High levels of cholesterol in the blood can cause a number of health problems, including an increased risk of heart disease. Changing your diet and lifestyle to reduce a high cholesterol level is essential for good health.

Cholesterol is important for a healthy body; it forms cell membranes and makes several hormones. Most cholesterol is made in the liver from saturated fats. If you consume more cholesterol (from meat, eggs, dairy products, seafood) the liver usually compensates by producing less. Cholesterol is carried in the blood by lipoproteins. High-density lipoproteins (HDLs) are the most efficient carriers, moving cholesterol safely between the liver and tissue cells. Low-density lipoproteins (LDLs) lose some cholesterol in the arteries, where it accumulates and forms fatty deposits called plaque. High levels of LDL cholesterol in the blood can cause a number of health problems, especially a greater risk of heart disease and stroke.

CHOLESTEROL LEVELS

In general, a desirable cholesterol level is between 180 and 200 milligrams per deciliter; borderline high is 200 to 240; above 240 is high. A test to determine the ratio of HDLs to LDLs is even more informative than an overall figure. The higher the HDLs the better. Not only do they keep cholesterol moving but they also clean up deposits left by the LDLs.

LOWERING CHOLESTEROL

A high-fat, low-fiber diet can increase blood cholesterol levels; to keep them down, choose low-fat foods rich in carbohydrates. Soluble fiber, found in oat and rice bran and many fruits, can reduce cholesterol because it binds with it in the large intestine, allowing it to be excreted.

Moderate amounts of alcohol, for example, one or two drinks per day, have been shown to boost levels of beneficial HDL cholesterol. Too much alcohol, however, can decrease HDL cholesterol and raise LDL levels.

It is important to prevent the oxidation of cholesterol in your body, which leads to free radical production. Stress is a major source of free radicals, so stress reduction is vital. Even mild exercise, such as walking or cycling, can raise HDL levels which in turn will lower the amount of LDL cholesterol in the blood. Use meditation techniques daily to help you to beat stress.

Cigarette smoking oxidizes LDL and limits HDL content, and compounds both cholesterol and smoking-related health problems.

THE ROLE OF CHOLESTEROL

Cholesterol is carried around the body by lipoproteins. The two main types are low-density (LDL), "bad" cholesterol, and high-density (HDL), "good" cholesterol. The difference between them is the amount of protein to cholesterol carried and their function. HDLs mop up the dangerous buildup of cholesterol that is deposited on artery walls by thwarted LDLs.

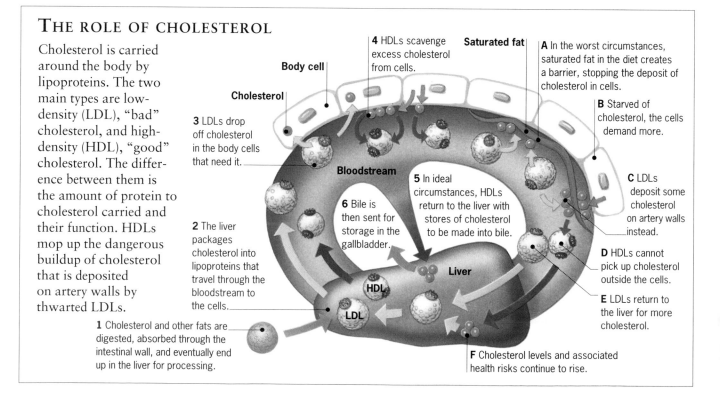

4 HDLs scavenge excess cholesterol from cells.

Saturated fat

A In the worst circumstances, saturated fat in the diet creates a barrier, stopping the deposit of cholesterol in cells.

Body cell

Cholesterol

B Starved of cholesterol, the cells demand more.

3 LDLs drop off cholesterol in the body cells that need it.

Bloodstream

5 In ideal circumstances, HDLs return to the liver with stores of cholesterol to be made into bile.

6 Bile is then sent for storage in the gallbladder.

C LDLs deposit some cholesterol on artery walls instead.

2 The liver packages cholesterol into lipoproteins that travel through the bloodstream to the cells.

Liver

HDL

D HDLs cannot pick up cholesterol outside the cells.

LDL

E LDLs return to the liver for more cholesterol.

1 Cholesterol and other fats are digested, absorbed through the intestinal wall, and eventually end up in the liver for processing.

F Cholesterol levels and associated health risks continue to rise.

STEP-BY-STEP RELIEF FROM HIGH CHOLESTEROL LEVELS

1 *CHOOSE LOW-FAT ALTERNATIVES.* Cut down the total amount of fat you eat so that no more than 30 percent of your daily calories come from fat. Saturated fat in particular should make up no more than 10 percent or less. Remember to check food labels for the fat content, both total and saturated.

HEALTHY ALTERNATIVES

Be aware of healthy options when dining out. Try to choose low-fat and high-fiber foods and, if possible, go for dishes that are steamed, grilled, or broiled rather than fried. If you are unsure, ask the waiter or waitress to guide you on the cooking methods and ingredients of the dishes.

2 *INCREASE SOLUBLE FIBER INTAKE.* There are two types of fiber: insoluble and soluble. Soluble fiber, found in oat and rice bran, barley, legumes, and fruit, can help lower cholesterol levels because it binds with cholesterol in the large intestine, allowing it to be excreted.

3 *REDUCE STRESS.* Stress increases cholesterol production in the body. It pays to learn some relaxation techniques and set aside time for doing exercise and for relaxation.

4 *WATCH YOUR WEIGHT.* Being overweight is one factor that contributes to high cholesterol. For people who are tring to lower weight and choles-terol, limiting total fat intake to 25 percent and saturated fat to 7 percent is even better than the advice above left.

Menu Ideas

There are many simple and economical ways to incorporate low-fat foods into your diet. You can substitute low-fat yogurt for mayonnaise, baked or boiled potatoes for chips, and white meat and fish for fatty red meat.

Breakfasts

For a filling, low-fat breakfast, try a bowl of oatmeal made with skim milk and topped with dried fruit, or combine some muesli, oat flakes, or bran flakes with chopped fresh fruit, such as apples, apricots, or peaches.

Lunches

Whole-grain bread with a chicken or turkey filling provides plenty of filling fiber and necessary protein. Pasta served with garlic and olive oil can help lower cholesterol. Serve it with a mixed green salad.

Dinners

Broiled chicken breast or fish, served with mixed vegetables and pasta or rice provide low-fat, high-fiber evening meals. Round off dinner with nonfat frozen yogurt to add a sweet treat to your day.

BAKED MACKEREL WITH RICE
Mackerel baked in foil with herbs, combined with rice and steamed vegetables, makes a healthy contribution to reducing and maintaining a healthy cholesterol level.

Mackerel offers a low-fat alternative to red meat and is also high in omega-3 fatty acids, which help lower cholesterol levels.

Carrots provide both fiber and beta carotene; the latter cleans up free radicals that can damage LDLs, causing them to deposit plaque.

Broccoli contains a good amount of fiber and is both low in fat and high in vitamins and minerals.

Snacks

Fresh fruit and low-fat crackers can help to stave off hunger pangs and ensure you don't snack on high-fat foods between meals.

Gluten-Allergy Plan

A food allergy is basically an overenthusiastic response by the immune system to a food substance. One of the most common food allergens is gluten, a protein in some grains. Replacing the allergenic foods should relieve symptoms.

The body's immune system is primed to respond to hostile foreign substances (antigens). Sometimes, however, it becomes sensitive to harmless substances, including some proteins in foods. The immune system's reaction to this harmless substance is called an allergic response. A relatively common food allergen is gluten, a protein found in wheat, rye, barley and oats.

Sensitivity to gluten also varies. Some people may be able to tolerate small amounts of gluten without any ill effects in the short term, although if they continue to consume foods that contain it, more serious consequences can develop.

The most serious disorder in which this allergy occurs is celiac disease; sufferers have a permanent intolerance to gluten, which gradually damages the small intestine.

People who suffer chronic yeast infections (see page 116), irritable bowel syndrome (see page 144), and skin problems such as eczema (see page 123), may also find that eliminating gluten from their diets will ease their symptoms.

In avoiding all those foods that contain gluten, it is necessary to find appropriate substitutes to ensure sufficient carbohydrate and fiber in the diet. Gluten-free breads and pastas are available in health food stores and pharmacies, although they are expensive. You may wish to make your own breads, or to seek alternative foods instead.

FOODS TO AVOID

Gluten is found in wheat, oats, rye and barley, which means that allergy sufferers must avoid a long list of foodstuffs and be diligent about reading food labels. They need to steer clear of foods that contain flour made from any of these grains, notably bread, cakes, pies, cookies, crackers, and anything made with bread crumbs. It means avoiding as well products in which flour may have been used as a thickener or filler, for example, gravies and sauces (ketchup is included), sausages, soup, and luncheon meats. Also on the list is any beverage made with malt, such as beer. Many breakfast cereals are eliminated, and pastas made with durum wheat. Foods that contain wheat starch, modified food starch, or hydrolyzed vegetable protein are also prohibited for people who are allergic to gluten.

FOODS TO INCLUDE

Those who suffer gluten allergies must compensate for the dietary fiber and complex carbohydrates on which they miss out. The main substitutes are potatoes, sweet potatoes, rice, and corn (including cornmeal and cornstarch). These can be used as staples and augmented by buckwheat (kasha) and legumes. To obtain the necessary fiber, select whole-kernel corn and rice products and eat rice bran, brown rice, and potatoes with their skins.

Fortunately, gluten-free flours, breads, and pastas are available. They are not widely distributed, but you can ask your local supermarket to order them for you. Look for bean, soy, and buckwheat flours and pasta made with Jerusalem artichokes.

SYMPTOMS OF GLUTEN ALLERGY

Unlike many other allergies, a gluten allergy does not involve the release of histamine from the body's cells. Instead, the damage is caused by the immune system reacting to a protein in gluten called gliadin. The reaction damages mucosa in the stomach, causing pain and a wide variety of symptoms that range from mental changes to pale, bulky stools to muscle wastage, and, in children who have the allergy, a failure to thrive.

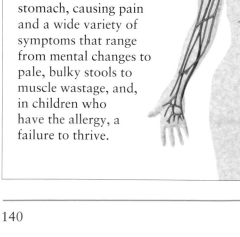

- **Possible neurological problems**
- **Mouth ulcers**
- **Possible cardiovascular problems**
- **Anemia**
- **Loss of appetite**
- **Chronic diarrhea**
- **Weight loss**
- **Abdominal distention**
- **No menstrual periods**
- **Fatigue**

STEP-BY-STEP FREEDOM FROM GLUTEN ALLERGY

1 SUBSTITUTES FOR FIBER
A gluten-free diet may mean that you lose out on some dietary fiber. Increase your intake of vegetables and fruits and eat whole-grain corn products, brown rice, and buckwheat.

2 SUBSTITUTES FOR CARBOHYDRATES
Use potatoes and rice as your carbohydrate-providing staples. Look for recipes that do not call for flour, such as cakes that use ground almonds instead.

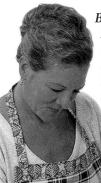

BAKING YOUR OWN
Baking gluten-free products yourself can be less expensive than buying those that are specially made.

3 READ THE LABEL
Always check the list of ingredients on food packaging carefully. Some of the most unlikely foods may contain gluten in their ingredients. Products such as salad dressings, stock cubes, soy sauce, gravy mixes, dry-roasted nuts, processed cheese spreads, beefburgers, pâtés, malted milk drinks, and soups are common culprits that can trip up the unwary buyer and lead to discomfort.

4 LOOK FOR THE SYMBOL
The international Gluten-Free Symbol is a crossed grain of wheat. This sign appears on cans and packages to indicate the product is free of gluten in all its forms. For a list of gluten-free products, contact the National Digestive Diseases Information Clearinghouse in Bethesda, Maryland.

Menu Ideas

The following plan gives you ideas for gluten-free meals, while ensuring that you obtain sufficient complex carbohydrates and fiber. If you are able to buy gluten-free breads and pasta you can include these in some meals.

Breakfast
Breakfast cereals that you can eat include cornflakes, puffed rice, and cornmeal porridge. You can replace toast with rice cakes. Buckwheat pancakes are also suitable; if you use a packaged mix, make sure it has none of the ingredients listed on the opposite page under "Foods to avoid."

Lunch
A baked potato or a brown-rice salad can form a nutritious base for lunch, with tuna, ham, chicken, or beans to provide protein. For a satisfying milkshake you can blend bananas with low-fat yogurt and honey.

Dinner
Try chili or grilled fish with rice. Remember to eat lots of greens and fruits to make up for the minerals and vitamins that you would normally obtain from grains.

LIGHT BREAKFAST
For a delicious and healthful gluten-free breakfast, serve a poached or boiled egg with rice cakes, mushrooms, and tomatoes.

Rice cakes or potato pancakes make excellent substitutes for toast.

A boiled egg provides high-quality protein and long-lasting energy.

Broiled tomatoes and mushrooms round out the nutritional content with substantial amounts of several vitamins and minerals.

Snacks
Fresh or dried fruit is always a good choice. Rice cakes can be used with various toppings in place of toast. Also, try unsalted, unsugared popcorn.

Lactose-Intolerance Plan

Many adults and some children, too, are unable to digest milk because they lack the enzyme lactase. The degree of intolerance varies, and there are many ways to get around it.

Intolerance to milk is very common, especially among adults, many of whom simply outgrow the ability to digest milk. About two-thirds of the world's population suffer some degree of lactose intolerance. The people most susceptible are those of African, Mediterranean, Asian, and Middle Eastern descent.

The typical symptoms bloating, gas, diarrhea, and abdominal cramping, usually set in within an hour of consuming milk or a milk product. When the lactose, or milk sugar, passes into the intestines undigested, it ferments there, causes gas, and gathers large amounts of water, leading to watery stools.

The degree of intolerance varies, with some people reacting to very small amounts of any dairy product and others having difficulty only when they consume large quantities.

An intolerance to lactose sometimes develops in people who have celiac disease (intolerance to gluten) or other intestinal condition in which the lining of the intestines becomes damaged and hinders lactase production. Once the other digestive problem is brought under control, the intolerance for milk usually disappears.

GETTING IT UNDER CONTROL

If you suspect that you have lactose intolerance but aren't certain, eliminate all milk and milk products from your diet for several days, then reintroduce them gradually in very small quantities. New research suggests that this approach may, in fact, help some people control their lactose intolerance without cutting out dairy products altogether. It is thought that the bacteria in the colon can adapt to occasional, small amounts of lactose.

Many people who have low levels of lactase can tolerate small amounts of milk—up to 240 ml (8 fl oz) a day—without experiencing discomfort. Some can eat yogurt with live cultures as well, because the bacteria in it break down part of the lactose. A number of people can also consume cheeses, especially aged ones, because they contain much less lactose than milk. An ounce of Cheddar cheese, for example, has less than 1 gram of lactose, compared to the 10 grams in an 8-ounce glass of milk.

Persons who are very sensitive to lactose have to avoid all forms of it. This means reading labels of packaged foods carefully for such words as whey, casein, lactose, nonfat milk powder, lactalbumin, and milk solids. It also means finding other products that can supply the necessary calcium. Many foods today are fortified with calcium to accommodate people who have difficulty with milk products. Among them are bread, waffles, soy milk, and orange juice. A package label will indicate the amount.

ALTERNATIVE FOODS

Several products are available to help people cope with lactose intolerance. Lactose-reduced milk is one; it contains less than 70 percent of the lactose found in regular milk. (Note: consuming lactose-reduced milk will not prevent a reaction if you are allergic to milk, characterized by wheezing, sneezing, and other typical signs of allergy.) There are also enzyme drops, found in pharmacies, that can be added to milk and enzyme tablets that can be taken before eating milk products. (The tablets are helpful if you are eating out and can't be certain what is in the dishes you order.)

THE EFFECTS OF LACTOSE INTOLERANCE

When the body fails to break down a substance, such as lactose (shown below), the failure of the system throws the body into disarray and leads to digestive problems such as diarrhea.

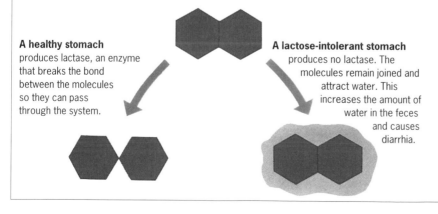

Lactose molecules are made up of two sections joined together, one of which is a glucose molecule. These pass from foods into the stomach where they are normally broken down.

A healthy stomach produces lactase, an enzyme that breaks the bond between the molecules so they can pass through the system.

A lactose-intolerant stomach produces no lactase. The molecules remain joined and attract water. This increases the amount of water in the feces and causes diarrhia.

STEP-BY-STEP RELIEF FROM LACTOSE INTOLERANCE

1 SUBSTITUTES FOR CALCIUM
Avoiding or reducing dairy products can reduce your calcium intake, so you need to include alternative sources in your daily diet. Two heaping tablespoons of sesame or sunflower seeds, 1 cup of red kidney beans, 3 sardines with bones, 50 g (1¼ oz) tofu, 5 figs, and a large serving of cabbage, broccoli, or spinach will each supply a good measure of calcium for your daily needs.

2 SUBSTITUTES FOR FAT
If you no longer eat any type of milk product, including cheese, your intake of saturated fats will be reduced. You may wish to replace some of these with unsaturated fats from oily fish and vegetable oils.

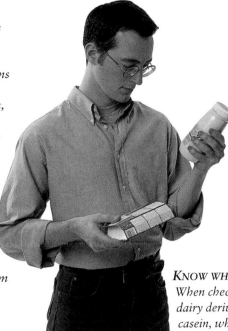

3 SUBSTITUTES FOR PROTEIN
A lactose-free diet may mean that you lose out on protein when you no longer eat cheese and dairy products, so replace these with extra servings of legumes, cereals, eggs, nuts, and tofu.

4 READ THE LABEL
Always check ingredients lists on food packaging carefully to make sure that no lactose foods slip through into your diet. This is particularly important in prepackaged meals, in which the ingredients may not be obvious from the name or look of the food.

KNOW WHAT TO LOOK FOR
When checking labels, look out for dairy derived additives like whey and casein, which are often added to sauces and even to some dairy substitutes.

Menu Ideas

These plans will help you gain sufficient calcium in your diet while avoiding lactose. Make sure you have at least one large glass of calcium-enriched soy milk each day. Soy desserts are also available from health food stores.

Breakfast
A whole-grain cereal with lactose-reduced milk, toast and marmalade, a boiled egg, and a glass of orange juice will start your day on a calcium and protein high.

Lunch
A salad made with lettuce, watercress, sunflower seeds, and canned salmon makes an excellent calcium-rich lunch. Similarly, hummus or sardines (with bones) on whole-grain toast boosts protein and calcium.

Dinner
Spiced lentils lend an exotic flavor to evening meals. Serve with brown rice or noodles and a spinach salad (for extra calcium). Follow with fresh figs for another calcium boost.

TOFU, PEPPER, AND BEANSPROUT STIR FRY WITH NOODLES
This dish provides a healthy source of protein and calcium (in the tofu), and carbohydrates (in the noodles).

Peppers are a rich source of vitamin C, while beansprouts provide a good supply of potassium.

Noodles provide a low-fat base to the dish and a reasonable serving of complex carbohydrates.

Snacks
Sunflower seeds, dried fruit, mixed nuts (including almonds), and dried figs are modest sources of calcium and are lactose-free.

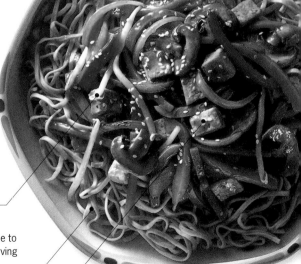

Tofu (bean curd) is made from soybeans and provides an excellent dairy-free source of protein and calcium.

Irritable-Bowel-Syndrome Plan

Poor diet is one of the main causes of irritable bowel syndrome (IBS). Most sufferers can relieve their symptoms with careful attention to their eating habits. Stress management is also important.

Irritable bowel syndroms (IBS) is a problem with the working of the smooth muscles of the intestines. These muscles normally propel food along by contracting and relaxing. Sometimes they lose this rhythmical movement and go into spasm, resulting in a variety of symptoms.

Although IBS and other bowel irregularities are not defined as serious illnesses, they can cause much discomfort and embarrassment to sufferers. They can restrict your lifestyle generally and make it hard to enjoy a normal social life.

THE CAUSES OF IBS
No one knows exactly what causes IBS but it is clear that there is no single or consistent cause. A variety of factors are usually involved. The most common of these are diet, such as a lack of fiber or a food intolerance, and stress, especially prolonged periods. IBS may also be triggered by gastric flu, gastroenteritis (a gastrointestinal infection), or a course of antibiotics or other drugs.

HOW CAN FIBER HELP?
A high-fiber diet can help to relieve and reduce some of the major symptoms of IBS. Fiber-rich foods such as whole-grain cereals, oats, beans, fruits, and vegetables absorb a lot of water (rather like a sponge). This water adds bulk to the feces, speeds the passage of food through the digestive system, and helps to restore the natural propulsive movements of the muscles. This produces bulky, soft stools that can be passed with less strain, relieving constipation and hemorrhoids.

If you tend toward constipation, avoid eating too much bran as this may cause gas and bloating. Instead, eat legumes and fruits, which contain soluble fiber. You should also drink at least eight cups of fluids a day.

If you are prone to diarrhea, avoid eating too many foods that stimulate uncontrolled bowel actions, for example, caffeine, alcohol, bran cereals, and dried fruit. If you are prone to flatulence, avoid gas-producing foods, such as beans and onions, and cut down on cruciferous vegetables (cauliflower, cabbage).

LIFESTYLE MEASURES
In addition to making adjustments to your diet there are also specific lifestyle changes you can make to help relieve symptoms. Establish regular bowel habits by visiting the lavatory at a similar time each day, but do not strain for a bowl movement. Always go to the bathroom whenever you feel the urge; never ignore it or try to hold on. Avoid laxatives unless your doctor advises their use because these do not encourage regular bowel movements.

As stress is known to provoke IBS, prioritize your workload, allowing time for relaxation. Exercise is not only a useful reliever of stress, it will also ease constipation by stimulating bowel movement.

Self-hypnosis and visualization have proved helpful in alleviating the symptoms of IBS when they have been used to help lower stress levels and promote a subconscious desire to feel healthy again.

It can help to replace coffee and tea with herbal teas such as chamomile and rosemary, which have an anti-spasmodic effect on the bowels.

A STOMACH'S HEALTHY BALANCE

There is a delicate balance of enzymes and acid in the stomach. A course of antibiotics, a bout of gastroenteritis, gastric flu, or even eating certain foods can affect this natural balance and cause problems in the breaking down and propelling of food.

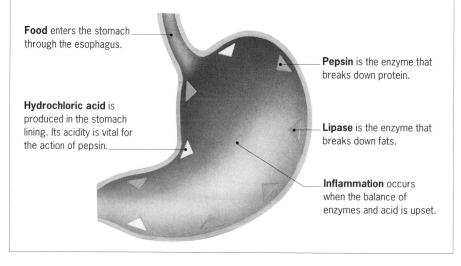

Food enters the stomach through the esophagus.

Hydrochloric acid is produced in the stomach lining. Its acidity is vital for the action of pepsin.

Pepsin is the enzyme that breaks down protein.

Lipase is the enzyme that breaks down fats.

Inflammation occurs when the balance of enzymes and acid is upset.

STEP-BY-STEP RELIEF FROM IRRITABLE BOWEL SYNDROME

1 EAT REGULAR MEALS
Eat regular meals and snacks—little and often rather than large infrequent amounts. Do not skip meals or leave gaps longer than three to four hours between eating. It is also important to eat slowly in a relaxed environment, to avoid taking in air while eating.

ENJOY EVERY MEAL
Do not skip meals, especially breakfast, or eat on the run. Sit down to your meals and take time to enjoy them.

2 INCREASE THE FIBER IN YOUR DIET
Soluble types of fiber, found in oat bran and fruit, are the most effective, helping to speed the passage of food through the digestive system and restore natural bowel movements.

3 REDUCE STRESS
Learn to manage your time in order to avoid overcommitting yourself, and take time out each day to relax and wind down. Find a form of relaxation that appeals to you, perhaps an aromatic bath or listening to music.

4 EXERCISE REGULARLY
Regular exercise will help combat stress; it can also help to stimulate bowel movements. Look at ways of introducing walking, swimming, or cycling on a regular basis into your life.

Menu Ideas

Including sufficient fiber in your diet promotes regular function of the intestines. Remember that you should tailor your meals to your own needs, avoiding foods that worsen your own particular symptoms.

Breakfast
A bowl of branflakes with added dried fruit (although not gas-producing prunes or dried apricots), or whole-wheat biscuits and milk, or a slice of whole-grain toast will boost your fiber levels at breakfast.

Lunch
Baked potato with baked beans and grated cheese or a whole-wheat pitta filled with a mixture of low-fat cheese, grated carrot, and raisins—either of these followed by a banana or pear would make an ideal lunch.

Dinner
Brown rice and lentils provide an excellent high-fiber base for an evening meal. These can be livened up with stir-fried chicken, vegetable stew or curry. A high-fiber dessert idea is fruit crumble made with rolled oats.

A LENTIL AND VEGETABLE STEW
This hearty stew, rich in fiber and a variety of vitamins, particularly vitamin C, makes an excellent warming autumn or winter meal.

Carrots and red peppers provide vitamin C, useful for building up your immune system, as well as providing fiber. By cooking them in a stew, you lose fewer of the vital nutrients because the nutrition-rich juices remain.

Snacks
Throughout the day you can boost your fiber levels with low-fat snacks of fresh or dried fruits and whole-grain breads, muffins, or crackers.

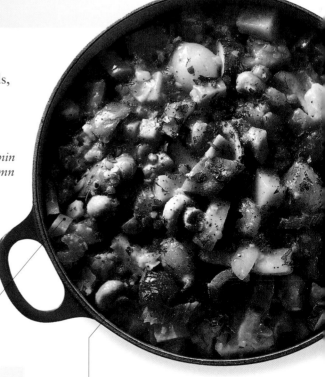

Lentils, like all legumes, are a good source of fiber, which promotes regular function of the intestines.

Anticraving Plan

Most people experience an almost uncontrollable urge for a certain food at some time. Although no one is sure why cravings occur, to beat unhealthy cravings it is necessary to change eating habits as well as the foods you eat.

Everyone occasionally has an irresistible urge for a certain food, but this does not constitute a true craving, which is an insistent desire that you can't ignore, even though satisfying it may be inconvenient or dangerous to health.

Some psychologists believe that one basis of cravings is the need for a carbohydrate-fat combination. Breast milk is sweet, so from infancy people develop a liking for sweet foods. Babies and young children also require a relatively high-fat diet to support rapid growth, but when they outgrow these needs, the craving for sweet and fatty foods may persist.

Sweet foods are often used as rewards or to give comfort during childhood. Adults with such experiences may turn to sweet things when they need cheering up or deserve congratulations for their achievements.

Research suggests that cravings occur just before menstruation begins because progesterone levels drop in the last week of the cycle. This affects the pituitary gland in the brain, which controls appetite. The metabolic rate goes up and the body burns calories faster, thus requiring more food to sustain it.

Cravings for pickles and other salty foods during pregnancy probably signal a physical need as well. A woman's blood volume doubles during this time and she needs extra sodium to maintain a proper fluid balance.

USEFUL NUTRIENTS

The most commonly craved food is chocolate. Chocolate evokes pleasurable feelings and emotions in many people; it also provides comfort and is a well-known antidote to feelings of depression. No one knows exactly why, but there are several theories.

Chocolate contains magnesium and iron, which the body may be craving. However, the amounts are small; you obtain more magnesium from two small bananas than a 50 g (1¾ oz) bar of milk chocolate, and more iron from two spears of broccoli.

Because chocolate has a unique combination of taste and texture it possibly produces a sensation in the mouth like no other food.

ADAPTING EATING HABITS

Foods that are strictly taboo invite disaster: as their desirability grows, you are more likely to eat them. Instead of banning a food altogether, it's generally better to permit yourself to eat anything in moderation. (The exception, of course, is when the food poses a danger to health, such as a very salty food for someone with hypertension.) You can also choose low-fat versions of especially rich foods that you like and try to find healthy substitutes that satisfy you.

If you do indulge a craving, eat only a small amount and enjoy your craved food slowly to prolong the pleasure without feeling guilty.

Base your meals on high-fiber starchy foods to satisfy your hunger. Studies have shown that starchy foods cause the brain to release serotonin and endorphins and thus improve mood and reduce fatigue.

If possible, eat five small meals a day to keep blood sugar levels steady. About 2 hours after a meal blood sugar levels drop (due to the action of insulin), energy levels flag, the brain's fuel supply falls, and hunger is experienced. Five small meals a day prevents the sugar level from dropping too far.

FOOD CRAVINGS

To help beat a food craving, try to isolate the particular characteristics of the food you crave and replace it with a healthier option whenever you feel your need for that food stirring.

CRAVED FOOD	CHARACTERISTIC	CHOOSE INSTEAD
Ice cream	Sweet, cool, and creamy comfort food	Low-fat ice cream or frozen yogurt, sorbet,
Chocolate candy	Sweet, smooth, and rich comfort food	Low-calorie chocolate, bananas
Cookies	Sweet crunchy or crispy food	Toast and low-sugar jam, low-fat cookies, apples,
Pie	Sweet and rich creamy or fruity food	pudding, custard, stewed fruit low-sugar jam or apple purée
Potato or corn chips	Savory crunchy or crispy food	Bread sticks, low-fat crackers rice cakes, popcorn

STEP-BY-STEP RELIEF FROM CRAVINGS

1 CHILDHOOD NEEDS
If a child develops a craving there are two possibilities to examine: poor diet and an emotional problem that needs attention. In the first case, if a child is continually offered an array of healthful foods, rather than chips or sweets, he will usually not pester you for the latter. In the second, if something is going wrong in his life, he may turn to certain foods for comfort, just as an adult would.

AN APPLE A DAY
.All children enjoy sweets, but it is possible to sow the seeds of an unhealthy food craving very young by giving a child sweet or fatty foods as a reward or a sign of love or comfort. Try to offer a healthy treat most of the time to provide balance.

2 ADULT NEEDS
Low mood and negative emotions can trigger food cravings. Sugary or starchy foods soothe and improve mood. When you are faced with a craving, it might help to examine your feelings and address the emotions behind it. Also, don't allow yourself to become overly hungry. The fatigue and depression caused by an empty stomach can lead to binge eating. As many cravings have at their core a psychological element, mind therapies, such as hypnosis, and relaxation techniques, like meditation, can also help.

3 BANNING THE GUILT
Cravings are natural and everyone gets them now and then. Chances are, if you allow yourself an occasional indulgence you will be less likely to develop cravings. If you give in to one, however, make the most of it by savoring it to the fullest.

Menu Ideas

To beat cravings, eat balanced meals with complex carbohydrates that provide sustained energy. Eat five meals a day, including mid-morning and mid-afternoon snacks to maintain blood sugar levels and prevent cravings.

Breakfast
Wheat flakes with milk and a sliced banana; fresh fruit, yogurt, and a bagel; or a bowl of oatmeal made with milk and topped with dried fruit will give you an excellent energy boost to begin the day.

Lunch
TK...TkA sandwich or a baked potato filled with cottage cheese, baked beans or chicken will boost carbohydrates
without piling on extra fat.

Dinner
TK,...TKA brown rice base makes an excellent evening meal when served with chicken or fish and a selection of vegetables. These dishes will be rich in carbohydrates, to help satisfy hunger pangs, and full of essential vitamins and minerals.

WHOLE-WHEAT TOAST WITH HONEY AND BANANA
A high-energy snack, such as toast and honey with banana slices, will maintain blood sugar levels and keep hunger at bay. This will help you avoid cravings during the day.

Banana is an excellent ingredient in simple snacks: it can help to maintain blood sugar levels by providing a slow release of energy.

Snacks
Rice cakes, fresh fruit, whole-grain crackers, air-popped popcorn, or a dried fruit bar all make super snacks to stave off cravings between meals.

Honey can help reduce cravings for highly sugary foods and whole-wheat toast can help maintain energy levels and reduce hunger pangs between meals

Quit-Smoking Plan

Smoking depletes the body's stores of several important vitamins, minerals, and antioxidants, leaving you more susceptible to fatigue and illness. If you're giving up smoking, you should eat to boost your body's overall nutritional status.

Smoking affects the natural defense system of your body by increasing the production of free radicals, highly unstable molecules that cause damage to cells, thus increasing the risk of cancer. It also depletes antioxidants, which block the action of free radicals. Although diet cannot undo all the damage caused by smoking, it can replenish your antioxidants.

The best source of antioxidant vitamins and minerals is the natural one: food. Supplements will not provide naturally occurring phytochemicals, substances with antioxidant properties that may also protect against various cancers and other degenerative diseases.

BEATING WITHDRAWAL

The first few weeks after quitting will be the most difficult, as you experience withdrawal symptoms and cravings for nicotine. You will have to cope with your physiological addiction to nicotine and overcome as well the need for a cigarette as a learned response to stress or social situations. In particular you may feel the craving for an oral fix—an urge to simply feel something in your mouth or between your lips.

AVOIDING WEIGHT GAIN

Many smokers experience weight gain when they quit. This is partly because nicotine raises the metabolic rate, so that while you are smoking you burn food more quickly, and also because ex-smokers start eating more, opting for a snack, when they might before have had a cigarette. The following tips can help you to avoid weight gain.

Keep your fat intake low, no more than 30 percent of your total calories. Cut down on fried foods, untrimmed cuts of meat, burgers, sausages, butter, margarine, whole-milk dairy products, cakes, chips, cookies, and chocolate. Instead of fatty snacks choose fresh fruit, toast, fruit bars, rice cakes, bread sticks, bagels, low-fat crackers, air-popped popcorn, yogurt, or dried fruit.

Obtain 55 to 60 percent of your daily calories from complex carbohydrate foods, such as bread, brown rice, legumes, fruit, and vegetables. And eat five to seven servings of fruits and vegetables each day for the benefit of their antioxidants.

Stay active to burn calories and avoid boredom. Walk instead of using the car for short journeys, use the stairs instead of the elevator, and do regular moderate exercise such as brisk walking or swimming (aim to be active three or four times a week).

PRACTICAL MEASURES

Nicotine addiction can be very powerful, and your willpower will be crucial in giving up. All your reserves of positive thinking will be called into play. You might find helpful one of the alternative therapies that have proved effective in quitting, including hypnotherapy and acupuncture. Relaxation techniques such as yoga, which concentrates on breathing, can also be beneficial. You could also try behavioral therapy—for example, giving yourself rewards for success or visualizing the negative effects of smoking, like the black-coated lungs, pictured at the left.

Maintaining your fluid levels will help alleviate cravings for a cigarette. Every time you desire tobacco, sip water, juice, or herbal tea. Chewing gum can also give you an oral fix without adding to your weight.

THE EFFECTS OF SMOKING

When you inhale cigarette smoke, particles of tar enter the lungs and attach themselves to the tissue.

The buildup of tar and its carcinogenic effect cause many respiratory disorders.

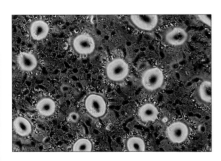

CIGARETTE SMOKE
For the most part, cigarette smoke is made up of tiny particles of tar. These are held suspended in a little water.

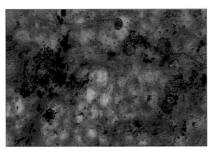

SMOKER'S LUNG
Here you can see the accumulation of tar deposits (the black areas) on the lung of a heavy smoker.

STEP-BY-STEP HELP TO STOP SMOKING

1 *REPLENISH YOUR ANTIOXIDANTS*
Every day, eat at least one food high in beta carotene (carrots, red peppers), vitamin C (oranges, broccoli), vitamin E (sunflower oil, peanuts) and powerful antioxidant minerals like selenium (whole grains, vegetables), zinc (bread, nuts, seeds) and copper (liver).

SATISFY YOUR ORAL CRAVINGS
Every time you crave a cigarette, substitute a healthy option, such as a glass of orange juice. It may also help reduce stress to take up a hobby or allow time each day to relax and read a favorite book or listen to music. Establishing any new routine can help break the habit as well as avoid trigger factors like boredom.

2 *AVOID WEIGHT GAIN*
Don't substitute sugary or high-fat snacks for cigarettes. Eat foods that are filling but low in calories, like whole-grain crackers, and limit your fat intake; avoid fried foods, whole-milk dairy products, cakes, and pastries. Burn off calories by climbing the stairs instead of taking the elevator, walking instead of driving, and doing moderate exercise.

3 *PRACTICAL MEASURES*
Avoid stress and keep a positive mindset by using relaxation methods. Ask your friends to help you by not offering you cigarettes, and identify the cues that trigger your craving so that you can avoid them. Satisfy your need for an oral fix by keeping fluid levels up, sipping healthy drinks, and chewing gum or munching on crudités.

Menu Ideas

After quitting smoking you need meals that are low in fat and high in vitamins and minerals, especially antioxidants. Such foods will help you keep weight off and aid your body in recovering from the harmful effects of smoking.

Breakfast
Eat something filling but low in fat. Avoid fried breakfasts in favor of whole-grain toast and cereals. Orange juice, fresh grapefruit, or fruit salad will provide vitamin C, an important antioxidant.

Lunch
Low-fat foods that are high in fiber will fill you up without being fattening. A good example is a whole-wheat pitta filled with tuna or hummus, accompanied by a green salad.

Dinner
High-fiber meals that are rich in antioxidant minerals and vitamins can be exciting, tasty, and even exotic. A meal of stir-fried prawns served with broccoli, onions, and carrots on a bed of noodles provides beta carotene, vitamin C, zinc, and selenium.

APRICOT MOUSSE
Try a tasty low-fat apricot mousse. It is high in fiber and an excellent source of vitamin C, beta carotene, and phytochemicals.

Apricots provide vitamin C and beta carotene, both powerful antioxidants.

Use fresh or dried apricots as a garnish to give extra tang, texture, and vitamins.

Snacks
Keep healthful snacks on hand that can provide antioxidants and a substitute for cigarettes. Citrus fruits provide vitamin C. Sunflower and sesame seeds are good sources of both zinc and vitamin E.

A fruit mousse can be as smooth or coarse as you like; you can add other ingredients to sharpen or sweeten the flavor or mix it with fruit salad or a warm fruit dessert.

Beating-the-Blues Plan

*What you eat can affect your mood as well as energy levels.
There is evidence that people may unconsciously choose foods that
change brain chemistry and put them in a better mood.*

Certain foods affect the production of neuro-transmitters (the brain's chemical messengers), one of the most important being serotonin. Low levels of serotonin have been linked to depression, sleeplessness, and fatigue. High levels can lift mood.

CARBOHYDRATES

People suffering from the blues often crave carbohydrates, consumption of which is known to affect serotonin levels. This is how it works: eating carbohydrates increases insulin levels, which in turn increase blood levels of the amino acid tryptophan. This enters the brain where it is converted into serotonin resulting in elevated mood (see diagram below).

PROTEIN FOODS

The mood-elevating effects of carbohydrates are strongest when they are eaten in combination with protein. Turkey, chicken, lean red meat, fish, dairy foods, and soy products are rich sources of protein and tryptophan. Eating them with a carbohydrate source is a good way to boost serotonin levels and mood.

FOLIC ACID

A deficiency of folic acid can exacerbate feelings of depression, as a doctor at McGill University in Canada discovered in 1993. In these tests people who were deprived of folic acid suffered from sleeplessness, forgetfulness, and irritability. Restoring folic acid caused the symptoms to disappear within a month.

Researchers found that the amount of folic acid contained in 150 grams (5½ ounces) of spinach resulted in a dramatic improvement in mood. Other folic acid-rich foods include liver, nuts, oranges, legumes, avocados, and fortified breads and cereals.

SELENIUM

Although an important mineral, selenium is required by the body in only tiny amounts. Evidence suggests that people with inadequate selenium are more likely to be depressed and tired. Increasing dietary selenium intake can help to reverse the effects.

Selenium is found in grains, seafood, fish, Brazil nuts, green leafy vegetables, and sunflower seeds.

The basis behind selenium's antidepressive properties is unclear, but it may be linked to its role as a powerful antioxidant (see page 148).

ZINC

Another mineral that helps to regulate moods and emotions is zinc. It is believed that some depressed people may respond well to small daily amounts. Good food sources include lean red meat, seafood, especially oysters, whole grains, beans, and fortified cereals.

VITAMIN C

Often regarded as the anti-stress vitamin, vitamin C can help to lift your mood when you are under emotional stress. It is found in broccoli, spinach and other green leafy vegetables, citrus fruits, berries, sweet peppers, and potatoes.

PRACTICAL MEASURES

Base your meals and snacks on nutritious carbohydrate foods such as potatoes, pasta, rice, bread, and fruit. Include at least two servings of protein-rich foods a day (for example, lean meat, dairy products, fish, legumes) to get enough tryptophan.

Some alternative therapies, such as Bach Flower remedies may help improve mood. Some studies show that mild exercise can be as effective as psychotherapy in the treatment of depression. Friends or professional counselors can also help.

SEROTONIN PRODUCTION

To boost levels of serotonin, it is important to have an adequate intake of carbohydrates. These trigger a reaction in the body that in turn causes a rise in serotonin in the brain and improves mood.

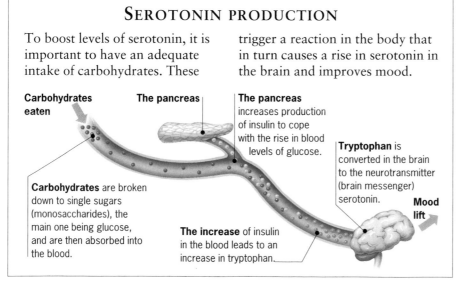

Carbohydrates eaten

The pancreas

The pancreas increases production of insulin to cope with the rise in blood levels of glucose.

Carbohydrates are broken down to single sugars (monosaccharides), the main one being glucose, and are then absorbed into the blood.

The increase of insulin in the blood leads to an increase in tryptophan.

Tryptophan is converted in the brain to the neurotransmitter (brain messenger) serotonin.

Mood lift

STEP-BY-STEP RELIEF FROM THE BLUES

GETTING OUT AND ABOUT
Lift your spirits by going on a picnic with a friend. The combination of sunlight, good company, and healthy food can work wonders for your mood.

1 BASE MEALS ON CARBOHYDRATES
Boost your levels of carbohydrates. Use potatoes, pasta, bread, brown rice, and fruit as the basis for your meals and snacks.

2 EAT TRYPTOPHAN-RICH FOODS
Protein-rich foods, particularly those high in tryptophan, will enhance the mood elevating effects of carbohydrates. Eat at least two servings a day of lean meat, dairy products, soy foods, or fish.

3 VITAMIN AND MINERAL INTAKE
Include plenty of dark green leafy vegetables for their folic acid and vitamin C content; citrus fruits and berries for vitamin C; and fish, oats, and whole-grain cereals and bread for their selenium content.

4 LIFESTYLE CHANGES
Adopting a modified diet shows the resolve to beat your depression. Maintain and add to this positive momentum by making other changes. Exercise and relaxation can help.

Menu Ideas

A mood-lifting diet should include plenty of green vegetables for folic acid, whole grains and seafood for selenium and zinc, and fresh fruit for vitamin C. Combining protein and carbohydrate in meals may boost your mood.

Breakfasts
Whole-grain cereals like muesli are a good source of selenium, high-fiber carbohydrates, and zinc. Complement them with fresh fruit for vitamin C, and nuts and seeds for more selenium to create a super start to your day.

Lunches
Pasta and chickpea salad provides carbohydrates and zinc. A fresh seafood and spinach salad is packed with protein, folic acid, zinc, and selenium.

Dinners
Serve garlic bread as a carbohydrate-rich starter, followed by chilli con carne with brown rice, to create a delicious protein and carbohydrate combination. Pasta with a seafood sauce like tomatoes and clams can achieve the same results. For dessert try rice pudding.

BRAZIL NUT AND VEGETABLE LOAF
As well as being low in fat and high in fiber, this dish is packed with complex carbohydrates, zinc, selenium, and vitamin C. Boost the mineral and vitamin content by serving this dish with potatoes and vegetables.

Brazil nuts are an excellent source of selenium and zinc, enhancing mood and providing antioxidants to fight free radicals at the same time.

Serve with vegetables or brown rice to boost your carbohydrate levels.

Snacks
Eat snacks that offer vitamins, minerals, and carbohydrates in a healthy form such as cereal, whole-grain toast, Brazil nuts, or sunflower seeds.

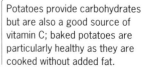
Potatoes provide carbohydrates but are also a good source of vitamin C; baked potatoes are particularly healthy as they are cooked without added fat.

Energy - Restoring Plan

Today's busy lifestyles can place huge demands on the body's energy levels. In order to restore and maintain energy levels so you can live your life to the fullest, be sure that you are eating the right amounts and types of food.

A prolonged period of stress can take its toll on energy stores. Weight-loss diets can also cause fatigue, as your metabolic rate slows down in an attempt to conserve energy.

B VITAMINS AND VITAMIN C
During times of stress it is especially important to take in extra amounts of the nutrients that support adrenal gland function (which controls production of many hormones) because the needs accelerate. They include vitamin C, vitamins B5 and B6, zinc, and magnesium. If these are lacking, lethargy and fatigue may result.

FREQUENT, SMALLER MEALS
A well-balanced and regular intake of vitamins and minerals is essential for energy production, so skipping meals or eating on the run can be particularly damaging to energy levels.

Breaking down your total food intake into smaller but more frequent meals, perhaps as many as six a day, achieves several important things. Blood sugar levels will be kept more stable, so your energy levels will remain high. You will avoid between-meal dips in energy, and your brain will receive a constant supply of glucose from the bloodstream. You will also avoid hunger pangs because blood sugar levels will be better controlled and your body will have a regular supply of food.

CARBOHYDRATES
People with high-stress lifestyles often rely on high-fat, high-sugar snacks in place of proper meals. Many fail to eat enough complex carbohydrates (starch), thus depleting levels of glycogen (stored carbohydrate), which leads to fatigue. It helps to snack on foods that are rich in complex carbohydrates, which provide a steady source of energy.

REDUCE STRESS LEVELS
A sense of helplessness and loss of control from excessive stress can make you feel fatigued before the day has even started. Quick lifts from caffeine-based drinks such as coffee or cola will have a mild stimulant effect but can also leave you feeling low once the effects have worn off. Avoid caffeine and try instead to employ relaxation techniques and follow the tips on this and the opposite page to replenish energy naturally.

LIFESTYLE APPROACHES
Getting eight hours of sleep a day is an effective way to stave off fatigue. If possible, get into a routine of going to bed early and rising early. You can also try the homeopathic remedy Arnica 6c to improve sleep (take one pill every 10 minutes for half an hour before going to bed).

Yoga enhances your breathing, so you take in more oxygen and feel energized. It also enhances circulation and strengthens internal organs.

Moderate exercise, even when you are tired, will help you to sleep better and boost your energy reserves.

THE ENERGY EQUATION

When your intake of carbohydrates (the most readily accessible form of energy) steadily matches the energy you expend, you achieve balance. If energy expenditure exceeds intake, the result is irritability, fatigue, and reduced mental alertness.

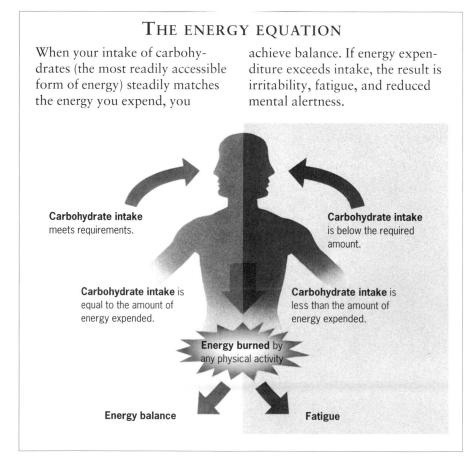

Carbohydrate intake meets requirements.

Carbohydrate intake is below the required amount.

Carbohydrate intake is equal to the amount of energy expended.

Carbohydrate intake is less than the amount of energy expended.

Energy burned by any physical activity

Energy balance

Fatigue

STEP-BY-STEP RELIEF FROM REDUCED ENERGY LEVELS

1 MAINTAIN VITAMIN LEVELS
A diet rich in B vitamins and vitamin C will help to restore energy levels by replenishing those used up in fighting stress. Foods high in these vitamins—fresh fruits and vegetables, whole-grain bread and cereals, nuts, and beans—can form part of a healthy diet with little need for complicated meals or major changes in shopping or cooking.

HEALTHY FOOD AT HAND
Keep your blood sugar levels up throughout the day by keeping healthy snacks at hand in your desk or work station.

2 EAT REGULAR SMALL MEALS
Regular, frequent meals help to raise your metabolic rate. Each time you eat, your metabolic rate increases approximately 10 percent. This is even more marked after eating a meal rich in carbohydrate and/or protein.

3 CARBOHYDRATE-RICH DIET
Complex carbohydrates found in pasta, potatoes, breakfast cereals, bread, beans, and cereal grains take longer to digest than low-fiber sugary foods. This means that they can make you feel satisfied longer and also produce a sustained rise in blood sugar, which helps to maintain energy levels. Rather than instinctively snacking on sugary foods, keep some dried fruit or nuts and seeds handy throughout the day.

4 REDUCE STRESS LEVELS
There are many techniques for relieving high stress levels. These can be as complex as a course in biofeedback—learning to control your brainwaves to induce relaxation—or as simple as taking time for yourself to enjoy a hobby or a pastime such as gardening or walking. Try to set aside a little time each day to escape from the pressures of day-to-day life.

Menu Ideas

Regular meals and mid-morning, afternoon and evening snacks that are high in carbohydrates and B vitamins, will help to boost your energy levels throughout the day. Aim to get at least half your calories from carbohydrates.

Breakfast
Try bran flakes with milk and fresh fruit, whole-grain toast with honey or a whole-wheat muffin and a glass of fruit juice. From these you can get the nutrients you need to start the day with an energy boost.

Lunch
A midday meal with a carbohydrate base, such as a sandwich made with whole-grain bead or a baked potato or rice dish, can be further comple-mented with cottage cheese, baked beans, or low-fat cheese.

Dinner
A high-carbohydrate meal consisting of a base of brown rice or whole-grain pasta can be enlivened with a chicken and vegetable sauce.

WHOLE-WHEAT PASTA
A chicken and vegetable sauce over whole-wheat pasta will provide vitamins and carbohydrates in a low-fat meal.

A sauce made with chicken breast, herbs, tomatoes, onions, and green vegetables provides protein and fiber.

Snacks
Use snacks to boost your food intake to six small meals a day. For an extra boost try a banana, toast with peanut butter, or a handful of dried fruit.

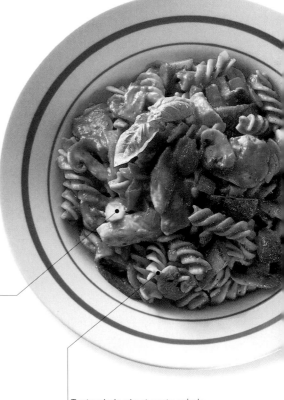

Tasty whole-wheat pasta spirals provide complex carbohydrates and B vitamins.

Memory-Improving Plan

Memory declines naturally with advancing age, but a diet rich in certain vitamins and minerals, coupled with a lifestyle tailored to maintain mental agility, may help to slow the decline and even improve memory.

Older people tend to absorb fewer nutrients because gastric juices decline with age. There is evidence that even a slight deficiency in certain nutrients can slow thinking and memory processes.

There are means of improving concentration, however, such as exercising the brain with puzzles or games, reading, participating in classes that require mental alertness, or memorizing poetry. Such activities are not only pleasantly diverting but also improve memory by stretching and testing it. Making special associations between names and places or events can help improve your recall.

Brain stimulation can also be increased by aerobic exercise such as jogging, swimming, and tennis.

Even mild deficiencies in the key nutrients involved in memory processes can impair memory. So even if a blood test is inconclusive, dietary changes to increase these nutrients may improve memory.

B VITAMINS

The B group of vitamins plays a vital role in regulating the brain's various functions, including memory.

A faulty memory is one of the main symptoms of thiamine deficiency, and some evidence suggests that improvements in memory occur after thiamine levels are increased. Thiamine is found in the outer part of grains, so when this is removed during refining most of the thiamine is lost. Thiamine is also found in nuts, beans, legumes, and meat.

Vitamin B_2 (riboflavin), B_3 (niacin), B_6 (pyridoxamine), and B_{12} are also implicated in memory processes, and rectifying deficiencies of these may help restore them. A lack of B_{12} can lead to memory loss, depression, and emotional problems.

Choline, a B vitamin found in lecithin (derived from eggs yolks and soybeans) has also been shown to boost declining memory. It is converted into a chemical messenger in the brain called acetylcholine, which transmits impulses from one neuron to another. Low levels have been measured in people with age-related memory loss and in sufferers of Alzheimer's disease.

Supplements may be necessary if it is not possible to get enough of these nutrients from food.

BETA CAROTENE

Recent tests at the U.S. Department of Agriculture's Human Nutrition Research Center found that people with adequate carotene levels did better on thinking tests than those with depleted levels. Beta carotene is found in yellow and orange fruits and vegetables, such as apricots, peppers, pumpkin, and carrots, and in green leafy vegetables.

MINERALS

Magnesium, essential for functioning of the nervous system, is involved in the memory process. Low levels may cause learning and memory problems.

Iron helps mental development during childhood. It is also needed throughout life to maintain the brain's healthy functioning. Iron deficiency can cause symptoms such as fatigue and impaired memory.

A deficiency of zinc can lead to a reduction in short-term memory and attention. Experiments have shown that normal healthy men and women who are marginally low in zinc perform poorly in memory tests. When their zinc levels are restored their mental performance improves.

MEMORY AND THE BRAIN

No one knows for sure where memory is stored in the brain. Many facets of memory are used every day, but following the path of a memory is difficult. People who have suffered damage to certain areas of the brain, such as the amygdala or the hippocampus, suffer a degree of memory loss. It is generally accepted, however, that the main storage area for memories is the cerebrum, particularly the cerebral cortex.

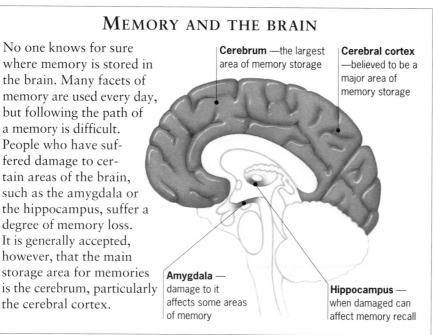

Cerebrum —the largest area of memory storage

Cerebral cortex —believed to be a major area of memory storage

Amygdala —damage to it affects some areas of memory

Hippocampus —when damaged can affect memory recall

STEP-BY-STEP PLAN TO IMPROVE MEMORY

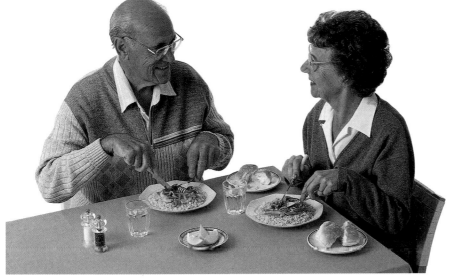

2 VITAMIN FOODS
*Choose vitamin-rich foods.
Riboflavin is found in dairy products and
nuts; niacin in potatoes, mushrooms,
seafood, and chicken; B_6 in potatoes,
chicken, spinach, and bananas; B_{12} in
dairy products, eggs, meat, and fish.*

3 BRAIN FOOD
*Increase your mineral intake.
Magnesium is found in nuts, seeds, green
leafy vegetables, bananas, and potatoes.
Good sources of iron include meat,
poultry, legumes, whole grains, and
green leafy vegetables; for zinc eat meats,
whole grains, seafood, and legumes.*

4 ALCOHOL AND MEMORY LOSS
*Drink alcoholic beverages in
moderation because chronically high
intakes of alcohol can damage brain
tissue and affect memory.*

EATING TOGETHER
*Sharing meals with a friend may help to
encourage healthy, regular eating
patterns and provide mental stimulation.*

1 SHARING MEALTIMES
*Nondietary changes include mental
stimulation, the most pleasant of which
may be simple mealtime conversation.*

Menu Ideas

When preparing unrefined foods, try steaming or stir-frying to preserve
their high mineral and vitamin content. Keep refined and processed foods
to a minimum because they are low in memory-restoring nutrients.

Breakfast
Add sunflower seeds to whole-grain
fortified cereal (for example, bran
flakes) and serve with milk. For a
more filling meal try poached eggs on
whole-grain toast. Alternatively, mix
milk, yogurt and banana for a
healthy breakfast drink.

Lunch
A toasted whole-wheat sandwich
filled with lean meat, tuna, or cheese
combined with tomatoes and spinach
contains nutrients needed to slow the
decline of memory. A good finish is
rice pudding and fresh fruit.

Dinner
Make casseroles with lentils or
chickpeas, both of which contain
choline. Alternatively, stir-fry
vegetables, chicken, and cashew nuts.

TUNA AND TOMATO SANDWICH
*A sandwich of whole-wheat bread or
rolls filled with a generous helping of
tuna, spinach, and tomatos contains all
the essential nutrients needed for
memory processes.*

Tomatoes add vitamins and
minerals, not to mention moisture
to a sandwich.

Whole-grain bread provides
thiamine and zinc.

Green leafy vegetables such
as spinach are rich in vitamin
A and iron.

Snack
For high-memory snacks, try
almonds, brazil nuts, and
sunflower seeds. For a sweeter
and protein-rich snack choose a
fruit-flavored yogurt.

Tuna offers riboflavin and zinc, as
well as protein. Another oily fish,
such as salmon, can be substituted.

GLOSSARY

Additive: man-made or natural chemical added to food to act as a flavoring, preservative, or coloring. Some cause side effects in susceptible people.

Amino acid: the basic building block from which the *protein* in muscles and other tissues is made.

Antacid: a substance that neutralizes excess acid in the stomach.

Antibacterial: a chemical that kills bacteria (minute organisms).

Antibiotic: an *antibacterial* chemical originally found in fungi. Many are now man-made.

Anticarcinogen: a substance that counteracts cancer-causing agents, such as *free radicals*. Many *antioxidants* have this property.

Anticoagulant: a chemical that thins the blood and reduces clotting. Some types help prevent heart attacks and strokes.

Antioxidant: a chemical that protects the body from the harmful effects of *free radicals*.

Antiviral: a chemical that kills viruses.

Beta carotene: a pigment that colors yellow-orange fruits and vegetables and most dark green vegetables. It is turned into vitamin A in the body, where it acts as an *antioxidant*.

Caffeine: a stimulant found in coffee, tea, chocolate, and some soft drinks.

Calcium: the most plentiful mineral in the body. Calcium is needed for nerve and muscle function, blood clotting, and metabolism.

Calorie: a unit of measurement used to calculate the energy stored in food. Protein and carbohydrates contain about 4 calories per gram. Fat yields about 9 calories per gram.

Carbohydrate: the principal energy food. Simple carbohydrates, or sugars, provide a ready source of energy that is quickly used up. Complex carbohydrates, as found in starchy foods, break down more slowly and provide the body with a steadier source of energy.

Carminative: food that helps the body to expel intestinal gas, relieving flatulence. Chamomile, rosemary, and peppermint are carminatives.

Cholesterol: a *lipid*-based substance vital for hormone production and the construction of cell membranes. May be deposited on the walls of blood vessels, causing high blood pressure and heart disease.

Crucifer: a vegetable of the Cruciferae family, including broccoli, kale, and cabbage, having cross-shaped blossoms and anticarcinogenic properties.

Diuretic: a substance that reduces water retention in the body by increasing the flow of urine. Foods with diuretic effects include asparagus, coffee, tea, onion, lemon, parsley, and peppermint.

Enzyme: a chemical catalyst vital to a wide range of bodily processes, such as the breakdown of food in digestion.

Fat: high-energy food. Some fat is vital to the body, but an excess can lead to disorders such as heart disease. Saturated fats can increase cholesterol levels in the body; mono- and polyunsaturated fats can reduce them.

Fiber: a mixture of substances that makes up plant cell walls. Insoluble fiber aids digestion and the passage of food through the gut; soluble fiber lowers *cholesterol* and helps regulate absorption of other nutrients.

Flavonoid: *antioxidant phytochemical*.

Folic acid: one of the B complex group of vitamins, vital for cell formation. Deficiency in pregnancy is associated with birth defects.

Food allergy: a condition in which the immune system reacts to a harmless component of the diet as if it were a disease organism.

Food aversion: a strong psychological reaction to certain foods.

Food intolerance: an inability to digest certain foods, usually because the appropriate enzyme is lacking. Food intolerance may lead to illness.

Free radical: a by-product of pollution, smoking, sunlight, and normal cell activity. Excess free radicals are linked to aging, heart disease, and cancer.

Gluten: a protein found in most cereals, which in some people can trigger a *food allergy* or a *food intolerance* complaint such as celiac disease.

Hormone: a chemical messenger that triggers many bodily processes. Some cancers are exacerbated by them; others are retarded. Some naturally occurring compounds can mimic them.

Lactobacillus: a type of bacterium often used to make yogurt. It is termed "friendly" because it can help to fight yeast infections and harmful bacteria.

Lactose: a type of sugar found in milk. Some people have a *food intolerance* to lactose and must avoid dairy products of any kind.

Lipid: a class of fat-based substances with a number of vital roles, including energy storage, hormone production, and the construction of cell membranes.

Lipoprotein: a fat-protein complex that transports cholesterol in the bloodstream. There are three types: high density (HDL), low density (LDL), and very low density(VLDL).

Mineral: a nonorganic element or compound that plays a vital role in the functioning of the body, often acting in concert with enzymes. Only tiny amounts of some minerals are needed.

Omega-3 fatty acid: an unsaturated fatty acid that cannot be manufactured in the body. Helps to thin the blood and relieve inflammation.

Phytic acid: a substance found in cereals and legumes that interferes with absorption of minerals. High amounts are present in raw bran.

Phytochemical: a plant chemical. Many of them have *antioxidant* properties.

Protein: a complex chain of *amino acids* that forms much of the structure and substance of living things.

Starch: a long chain of sugar molecules used by plants for storing energy. A complex carbohydrate.

Sugar: basic carbohydrate unit, the main source of energy in plants and animals.

Trans fatty acid: a type of fatty acid, similar to saturated fat, that has potentially harmful effects on the heart.

Vitamin: a naturally occurring substance that plays a part in all cell activities. Some vitamins can be made in the body from other elements, but most can be obtained only from food.

INDEX

ACKNOWLEDGMENTS

Carroll & Brown Limited would like to thank

Sharon Freed
Cancer Research Campaign
British Fertility Society
Institute of Research into
    Complementary Medicine
Department of Health, London

Editorial assistance
Hilary Sagar
Simon Warmer

Design assistance
Mari Hughes
Gilda Pacitti
Matt Sanderman
Jonathan Wainwright

Photograph sources
8   J-L Chermet/SPL
9   SPL
11   Lawrence Berkeley
     Laboratory/SPL
12   David Scharf/SPL
17   Tony Stone
18   SPL
30   Simon Fraser/SPL
34   (top) NIBSC/SPL
     (bottom) Biology Media/SPL
38   ZEFA
42   Department of Clinical
     Radiology, Salisbury District
     Hospital/SPL
43   SPL
86   Andrew Syred/SPL
92   American Academy of
     Environmental Medicine
96   Alfred Pasieka/SPL
97   Alfred Pasieka/SPL
102 Biozentrum/SPL
104 Jean-Perrin/CNRI/SPL
104 Department of Nuclear
     Medicine, Charing Cross
     Hospital/SPL
106 Professors P. Motta & F.
     Carpino, University 'La
     Sapienza', Rome/SPL
115 Alfred Pasieka/SPL
116 Dr Kari Lounatmaa/SPL
117 Andrew Syred/SPL
118 Breast Screening Unit, King's
     College Hospital, London/SPL
120 SPL
124 (left) Mike Devlin/SPL
     (right) CNRI/SPL
127 CNRI/SPL
132 (top) CNRI/SPL
132 (bottom) Wellcome Dept. of
     Cognitive Neurology/SPL
134 Alfred Pasieka/SPL
148 (left) Andrew Syred/SPL
     (right) Dr Clive Kocher/SPL

Medical illustrators
Sandie Hill
Paul Williams

Illustrators
Anna Koska
Vanessa Luff
Christine Pilsworth
Sam Thompson
Sarah Venus
Ann Winterbotham

Photographic assistants
Mark Langridge
M-A Hugo

Hair and make-up
Kym Menzies
Bettina Graham

Picture researcher
Sandra Schneider

Food preparation
Maddalena Bastianelli
Eric Treuillé

Research
Steven Chong

Index
Joel Levy

Note
Metric and imperial measures are given
throughout except when calculating measures
of nutrients, which are given in metric only.